Discoveries of Medically Themed Media

Lexington Studies in Health Communication

Series Editor: Leandra H. Hernández and Kari Nixon

National and international governments have recognized the importance of widespread, timely, and effective health communication, as research shows that accurate, patient-centered, and culturally competent health communication can improve patient and community healthcare outcomes. This interdisciplinary series examines the role of health communication in society and is receptive to manuscripts and edited volumes that use a variety of theoretical, methodological, interdisciplinary, and intersectional approaches. We invite contributions on a variety of health communication topics including but not limited to health communication in a digital age; race, gender, ethnicity, class, physical abilities, and health communication; critical approaches to health communication; feminisms and health communication; LGBTQIA health; interpersonal health communication perspectives; rhetorical approaches to health communication; organizational approaches to health communication; health campaigns, media effects, and health communication; multicultural approaches to health communication; and international health communication. This series is open to contributions from scholars representing communication, women's and gender studies, public health, health education, discursive analyses of medical rhetoric, and other disciplines whose work interrogates and explores these topics. Successful proposals will be accessible to an interdisciplinary audience, advance our understanding of contemporary approaches to health communication, and enrich our conversations about the importance of health communication in today's health landscape.

Recent Titles in this Series

Discoveries of Medically Themed Media: Pediatric Patients and Parents' Journeys of Sense-Making.

The Rhetoric of Breast Cancer: Patient-to-Patient Discourse in an Online Community.

Discoveries of Medically Themed Media

Pediatric Patients and Parents' Journeys of Sense-making

Heather A. Stilwell

LEXINGTON BOOKS
Lanham • Boulder • New York • London

Published by Lexington Books
An imprint of The Rowman & Littlefield Publishing Group, Inc.
4501 Forbes Boulevard, Suite 200, Lanham, Maryland 20706
www.rowman.com

Unit A, Whitacre Mews, 26-34 Stannary Street, London SE11 4AB

British Library Cataloguing in Publication Information Available

Library of Congress Cataloging-in-Publication Data

Names: Stilwell, Heather, author.
Title: Discoveries of medically-themed media : pediatric patients and parents' journeys of sense-making / Heather Hamilton-Stilwell.
Description: Lanham : Lexington Books, [2017] | Series: Lexington studies in health communication | Includes bibliographical references and index.
Identifiers: LCCN 2017044719 (print) | LCCN 2017044253 (ebook) | ISBN 9781498551991 (Electronic) | ISBN 9781498551984 (cloth : alk. paper)
Subjects: LCSH: Communication in pediatrics. | Communication in medicine. | Mass media in health education.
Classification: LCC RJ26.3 (print) | LCC RJ26.3 .S75 2017 (ebook) | DDC 618.920001/4—dc23
LC record available at https://lccn.loc.gov/2017044719

∞™ The paper used in this publication meets the minimum requirements of American National Standard for Information Sciences—Permanence of Paper for Printed Library Materials, ANSI/NISO Z39.48-1992.

Printed in the United States of America.

Contents

Preface

The concept of making sense of a medical experience and its plethora of challenges was not on the horizon of my mind's eye when I became a mommy, but without me realizing it, I set out on a sense-making venture with my precious little girl that night as she was born. As our other two children were born, they, too, have had to make sense of our crazy, "normal" life. This book is truly a labor of love built on my own experiences of fumbling around in hopes of knowing how to help them construct an understanding of the medical diagnoses that have become a very real part of our daily lives. And in all honesty, I wrote portions of this book while sitting next to my girl's hospital bed as we navigated the sense-making of new concerns and fearful procedures.

In addition to my daughter, you are about to meet 13 amazing children undergoing craniofacial, neurological, or neurosurgical treatment. Their expectancy of pain and sensitivity to anxiety has had considerable and concurrent effects (Kennedy, Moore, Peterson, Katzman, Vermani, & Charmak, 2011). Much of these children's struggles come from navigating the pain and anxiety coupled with the uncertainty of their treatments and what challenges tomorrow may hold—all things I have witnessed firsthand. It is through listening to their stories that great insight about their information needs and what tools can best help them and children like them is gained. In fact, medical narratives add depth to aspects of communication and behavior that are often left as pages unturned (Harter, 2013).

One of the most significant and unique ideas to come from this book is the notion of medically themed media as an information source and sense-making tool. As the children's stories explain, much of the available information about their diagnoses and treatment approaches is not delivered in an age-appropriate manner for children but rather geared toward adults.

There is a need to bridge mediated coping behaviors and young children's medical experiences. This is an imperative area of research as children's media and its influential role continues to grow and impact society.

Technological advancements have required scholars to look beyond traditional platforms of print, radio, or television and include multiple on-screen formats, including the Internet and smart phones. However, while most research centers on how children use media, the continuing evolution within children's media beckons how mediated narratives can be used to have a positive impact on children in some of their most vulnerable moments as they experience various medical situations. What you are about to read will build the case for medically themed media, a phrase that delineates popular books, music, video games, television shows, videos, and movies that include material, specifically narratives, dealing with medical events, issues, and experiences.

Medically themed media can be characterized as having prosocial content that seek to endorse and further socially beneficial behavior within a society (Lovelace & Huston, 1983). Audiences' exposure to a child's visit to the hospital, a doctor's description of a procedure, or family members' experiences with observing their loved one's medical journey are all examples of medically themed media that incorporate important and impacting lessons into narratives specifically related to medical situations. These media can be geared toward specific age groups and audiences further diversifying their content and effectiveness. This book's primary focus will center on medically themed media appropriately fashioned for use with young children experiencing a variety of difficult and traumatizing medical procedures.

The seeds of this study were originally planted during my first semester of PhD coursework. With the permission of faculty members who only knew me by my admission's paperwork, I was allowed to take the course, *Children and the Media*—a course not typically offered to incoming students. The course was not offered again during my time in the program, but it lay a foundation for what is now my passion of research. I am so grateful for the opportunity as it truly changed the trajectory of my doctoral studies.

Because stories help to humanize medicine (Harter, 2013), my research employed an ethnographical approach. Merriam (2002) maintained that ethnographies are basic interpretive qualitative research; additionally Tracy (2013) noted that they seek to describe people and their cultures. This book takes a reflexive narrative approach making use of hermeneutic phenomenological ideals to understand the medical experiences of children and their unique perspectives of them, including various means of communication that have helped or could help them in navigating the difficult and scary situations related to their medical situations.

The goal was to gain in-depth knowledge through the voices of these children and their families. I was not the outside researcher looking in on the stories of the 14 pediatric patients described in this book; my own experiences as a "medical mama" provided a unique position within which to discover and share these children's stories. My personal experience also added to the validity of this research, especially in that I brought greater access to, genuine interest in, and an intimate knowledge related to these children and their experiences (Adler & Adler, 1997; Beyer, 1992; Denzin & Lincoln, 1994). Given my association with the group being studied, reflexive insights helped bring about the emotionally rich narratives we will learn from; however, we will also see that through the telling of their stories so many of the children and their families discovered things about their journey that had not yet been explored and realized. Indeed, ethnographic research provides a powerful and intimate way of discovery. It is my hope that you, too, are moved to new discovery as you read their stories.

—Heather A. Stilwell, PhD

Acknowledgments

This book is a result of so much support as friends, mentors, and family championed me along the way. I am beyond thankful to my husband, Steve, for going this journey with me; you know research is the beat of my heart and your selfless support means so much. This book would not be complete without your gentle prodding to keep going. Reagan, Rhyan, and Jordan, I am so glad you call me Mom. You each teach me daily and make me better; I am grateful for your desire to make sense of and construct an understanding of who God created you to be. I also thank the rest of my family, especially my parents, John and Sue Hamilton, for giving me encouragement and support along the way.

My interest in scholarly research was birthed as an undergraduate student sitting in Dr. Paul Creasman's research methods course. Paul, you whet my appetite for scholarship and I am grateful for your mentorship over the years. I am also extremely grateful for the insight provided by the faculty at Regent University's School of Communication and the Arts. Dr. William Brown, Dr. Benson Fraser, and especially Dr. John Keeler, thank you for believing in this project and encouraging me throughout it.

I cannot thank the parents and children who opened their homes and lives to me enough. Without you this research would not have been possible. Each family provided such rich insight into what a journey of making sense of difficult medical challenges entails. I am so thankful for your honesty and willingness to be vulnerable. This book is for you and all the families you represent. Next time I will bring tissue! Additionally, this project would not have been possible without the help of Dr. Pedro Sanchez and Dr. Sheryl Lewin who believed in it and helped me with initial recruitment of participants.

Lastly, I am beyond grateful for the support of the many nurses, nurse and staff assistants, child life specialists, physician assistants, therapists, doctors, surgeons, anesthesiologists, special education teachers and aides, administrative assistants, and EMTs during some very trying times of my own girl's medical journey. Thank you to all the special medical professionals who give of themselves daily to make these little ones' lives better. It is the little things you do (e.g., going to the hospital gift shop to buy a stuffed animal because one was forgotten in the rush to the emergency room, decorating a bandage to make it look more like a sticker, or pretending to do vitals on a stuffed animal first) that do not get charted but make a huge difference. Without your sensitivity and a desire to create a safe space, the sense-making journey for these little ones would be next to impossible.

Introduction

Anything but the Expected

Fear was her regular response to a perceived threat, and her experience during doctor visits and procedures supported what has already been discovered: that one of the most common childhood phobias is medical events (Du, Jaaniste, Champion, & Yap, 2008; King, Heyne, Gullone, and Molloy, 2001). As Reagan has grown there have been very few moments of reprieve from unfamiliar doctors, nurses, procedures, equipment, and unfortunately discomfort or pain. She has known no different from the moment she was born.

Moments after Reagan was born, all my expectations seemed to crumble. An eight-pound baby with a very full head of hair was placed in my arms after nurses whispered among themselves while taking multiple Apgar scores. I sensed something was not right, but no one would say. And who was I to question at that moment; I was a first-time mother after all. Yet within hours of her birth, Reagan would begin to experience medical procedures. My fears were confirmed as a neurosurgeon gave us the diagnosis of craniosynostosis, a condition carrying craniofacial anomalies and often one or more syndromes.

By six months of age, Reagan would undergo a ten-hour neurosurgery to reconstruct craniofacial anomalies and spend a week in the Pediatric Intensive Care Unit. It would take her nearly a year to grow a full head of hair again—one that would cover the zigzagged incision stretching from ear to ear. Her infant oblivion to people's stares saved the then-innocence of her soul; however, as she neared toddlerhood confusion and frustration set in with every doctor's visit or medical procedure. By this time we had genetic test results that further complicated the road ahead.

As a parent, I felt helpless. How could I comfort her? It was nearly impossible to reason with a child so young. However, like the beginning streaks of a morning's sunrise hope poked through our clouds of frustration during the afternoon of one admission—an admission that would prove to be nearly five weeks long. As our nurse was reviewing our records and helping us get situated in our room, she gave three-year-old Reagan a yellow stethoscope. This stethoscope became the one the nurses and doctors would use. We played with it, pretended to listen to her dolly's heart, and took turns being the doctor who listened to the other's lungs. This stethoscope symbolized a sense of ownership regarding her situation; her emotions about the situation mattered. While this reality was not directly communicated, Reagan's behavior proved that a simple gesture, such as the giving of a stethoscope, could indirectly impact a situation.

As time went on, Reagan experienced more hospitalizations. They remained traumatizing. Aspects of her experiences were easier, partly because of familiarity; additionally, she began to identify with mediated narratives that subliminally provided information, encouraged bravery, and instilled notions of hope and the value of her life in spite of the present difficulty—all critical aspects of communicating resiliency to a small soul.

The art of overhearing truths is perhaps one of narratives' greatest strengths. By it readers are impacted through a message that is not specifically addressed to them (Craddock, 2002). This may be most true of children's narratives because as children rely on how a story is rhetorically framed, the narratives have the opportunity to help children make sense of their experiences. Brenda Dervin (1983) developed a sense-making model for use within ethnographic research; it considers how individuals use their observations of themselves, others, and life events to construct ideas of reality that then guide communicative behavior. Mediated narratives provide individuals with the opportunity to bypass the element of live in-person dialogue with other people and go through the sense-making process individually. Brown, Stacey, and Nandhakumar (2008) found that while "much sense is shared, [people] are strategically motivated to determine their own highly personal interpretations of what has occurred" (p. 1052). Narratives are indeed persuasive in how meanings are understood; sense-making of individual micro-level stories help to make sense of organizational macro-level stories (Brown et al., 2008). Furthermore, mediated narratives with medical themes provide the opportunity for children to internalize these indirectly communicated truths and transform them into a powerful personal storyline of bravery, hope, and value.

MEDIA'S HOPEFUL POSSIBILITY

Medically themed media capitalize on this ability to rhetorically posit notions of characteristics leading to resiliency within the mediated lives of socially significant characters portrayed in popular books, music, video games, television shows, videos, and movies that include material, specifically narratives, dealing with medical events, issues, and experiences. Given the impressionability of children (Hurst, Corning, and Ferrante, 2012), medically themed media are an excellent information resource to encourage understanding of medical procedures, teach coping tactics, and encourage resiliency concerning the value that life holds in spite of the challenges of various medical journeys. Coles (1990) noted, "Children try to understand not only what is happening to them but why; and in so doing that, they call upon the religious life they have experienced, the spiritual values they have received, as well as other sources of potential explanation" (p. 100). In these sources, there is an attempt to build a bridge between the unexpected and a desired hope.

The framework of these media and their unique rhetorical manner impact children's ability to make sense of their difficult experiences. Bettelheim (1975/2010) poignantly stated:

> [A child] can achieve this understanding, and with it the ability to cope, not through rational comprehension of the nature and content of his unconscious, but by becoming familiar with it through spinning out daydreams—ruminating, rearranging, and fantasizing about suitable story elements in response to unconscious pressures. By doing this, the child fits unconscious content into conscious fantasies, which then enable him to deal with that content. It is here that fairy tales have unequaled value, beause they offer new dimensions to the child's imagination which would be impossible for him to discover as truly on his own.

Specifically concerning children journeying through pain, mediated narratives have the opportunity to meet their needs and help them make sense of their experiences. Truths effectively communicated via narratives are important in the process of children making sense of their experiences and self-worth. This is because children's personal narratives are also rhetorical. Individual narratives are persuasive in how meanings are understood and legitimized at the organizational level (Brown et al., 2008). As children grow, they are seeking to figure out who they want to be as a person, what their future could entail, and the type of person with whom they might spend their life (Warren, 1997).

Even today, at the young age of seven, Reagan references medically themed media in an attempt to understand her experiences. In them, she is able to *overhear* strategies for resilience and truths that most likely would otherwise never be understood. An example of such is recalling how a character from a book or show remains brave before receiving a vaccination; whenever Reagan finds herself in a similar situation of being poked by a needle, she recites the words the character says about thinking something happy and focusing on the temporal nature of the discomfort. In this, she tries to remain brave herself. However, her struggles are often far more complex than coping through one poke. The unpredictable nature of her journey has often left us searching for additional resources that can continue indirectly communicating hope and value while helping her make sense of such unexpected and difficult circumstances. And we are not alone in this quest. The next chapter introduces 13 other children who with their families are also on a similar sense-making quest for resilience.

Chapter 1

Stories of Resilience

Within a healthcare context, the realizing and use of stories as part of treatment, and the conveying of one's journey through story can help others better understand the complexity of a patient's situation. The busyness of the medicine business often drowns out the richness of the narratives playing out, whether they are among patients and patients' families, families and medical personnel, or both. Hearing raw emotions as children recount their medical experiences and share their unique perspectives helps to humanize the often sterile and intangible concept of medicine (Harter, 2013). It is the powerful rhetoric within an ethnography that provides this insight and through the sharing of private stories that public impact can be made (Carabaş & Harter, 2005).

You are about to meet children from Alberta, Canada, and Southern California; each of them has either a neurologic, neurosurgical, or craniofacial diagnosis. While this is a niche group of diagnoses, there is a diversity and complexity of medical care represented. In addition to hearing from them, we will gain insight into their experiences as a result of drawings they did while I spent time with them; the meaning that comes from their artwork is profound.

Before you meet them, first allow me the opportunity to explain my ethnographic approach. I desired to make a compassionate space for the overwhelming threads of what may feel as an untamable fabric within these children's lives. For many, their stories are still unfolding and can be difficult to fully articulate and hard to listen to and understand (Frank, 1995). Often times we herald what Frank (1995) called the "restitution" story that describes the difficult medical journey that results in successful treatment and healing; likewise, patients who are in the midst of treatment tell the "quest" story as a means of framing their journey in hope for reaching healing. Yet, so many families' stories are filled with the messiness of unknowns and disheartening twist-and-turns along the medical journey. The children are unsure and parents question how to best help their children. This "chaos" narrative that is less told is in such great need of assistance and simply being heard (Frank, 1995).

I wanted to hear each child's story and understand their raw emotions that come with the fearful procedures; I wanted to grasp this information while ensuring that the struggle of these children and their families was not misrepresented. To do this, I used elements of Brenda Dervin's (1983; 1992; 2003a, b, c; 2008) Sense-Making Methodology and Micro-Moment Time-Line Interviewing (see Appendix A) along with a drawing method purported by Liamputtong and Fernandes (2015) that uses prompts to encourage children to draw and then reflect on their art (see Appendix A).

The children's drawings (see Appendix B) underlined the value of the stories told by the children participating in this study. They provided insight into the multimodal ways in which children narrate their experiences and construct meaning. The combination of interviewing and drawing, in addition to observation, helped to break down barriers and make the children more comfortable while allowing powerful space for their insights and emotions about medical experiences and coping techniques to be expressed.

This group brings a unique opportunity to gain insight into a largely understudied population of diagnoses and provides a greater understanding of the ways pediatric patients overall construct an understanding of medical experiences; much of the research concerning pediatric patients to date has centered in oncology communities. I hope that you are able to feel a bit of their plight but also recognize their strengths. May we not merely separate them as a collective group different from the majority of a society out of the assumption that they are suffering victims (Parsloe, 2015; Chew, 2008; Fine & Asch, 1988; Zola, 1993). Instead, each of the participant's stories below teach us about the value of *each* life and how shared existence with caretakers, family members, doctors, nurses, therapists, etc. is beneficial to the greater community.

ALBERTA, CANADA INTERVIEWS

A few years ago, one of my daughter's neurosurgeons, who was from Alberta, Canada, and very familiar with the renowned Stollery Children's Hospital in Edmonton there, suggested I look into joining an independent pediatric neurosurgical online support group for parents, which was started by a handful of moms with children undergoing neurosurgical care at the Stollery. While the majority of the group's members are from the Alberta area, I found the group to be very inclusive and full of great resources. It is through my connections

Table 1.1 Participants Undergoing Craniofacial, Neurological, or Neurosurgical Treatment

Name	*Gender*	*Age*	*Geographical Residence*	*Diagnosis*
Bethany	F	11	Alberta, Canada	Grade-1 pilocytic astrocytoma brain tumor & posterior process syndrome
Brooks	M	12	Southern California	Unilateral microtia atresia
Frankie	F	13	Alberta, Canada	Cleft lip and palate anomalies & developmental delay
Hannah	F	6	Alberta, Canada	Treacher Collins Syndrome
Jacob	M	3	Alberta, Canada	Cerebellar hypoplasia, bronchomalacia, & cardiac defects
Kyler	M	8	Southern California	Bilateral microtia atresia
Leslie	F	7	Southern California	Cerebral Palsy
Nadia	F	7	Alberta, Canada	Frontal lobe hydrocephalus & developmental delay
Nathan	M	13	Alberta, Canada	Epilepsy & developmental delay
Peter	M	5	Alberta, Canada	Cleft lip and palate
Reagan	F	6	Southern California	Craniosynostosis, hydrocephalus, & chiari malformation
Taylor	F	13	Alberta, Canada	Craniosynostosis & chiari malformation
Victor	M	3	Southern California	Cleft lip and palate
Wyatt	M	4	Southern California	Spina bifida, hydrocephalus, & chiari malformation

Note: Age is at time of interview.

with a couple of the moms in this group that I further met other families who agreed to share their stories.

With just two weeks before Christmas, the families in the Alberta area graciously opened their homes to me and so I made quick arrangements and traveled north of the United States' border for a week's stay. As my plane approached the airport, I could see nothing but white. Snow blanketed the city famous for its oil with temperatures hovering around zero degrees Fahrenheit. Because of the weather, interviews were conducted in the families' homes most often over hot cups of tea. Only one family was unable to meet in person during my time in Alberta; I followed-up with the child and her mother via FaceTime, Apple's online video chat. The following introductions represent eight amazing and strong children from six remarkable families.

Bethany

The sun was shining brightly and gleaming off the snow-lined streets as I drove to meet Bethany and her family at their home that Saturday morning. George, Bethany's father, was out front shoveling the driveway and sidewalk. He welcomed us and said Paula, his wife and Bethany's mother, and Bethany were waiting inside. Eleven-year-old Bethany was sitting on the living room couch covered in a blanket. She was reluctant to talk with me; although, it was a better option than cleaning her playroom.

We sat down at the kitchen table and began talking. Paula offered me tea and cookies as we talked. Bethany began by telling me about her love for recreational basketball, ice skating, and skiing. She described herself as "sporty" just like her favorite television show character, Maddie, from Disney Channel's *Liv and Maddie* (personal communication, December 19, 2015). Bethany also had a few favorite books: *Love You Forever*, a story about the relationship between a mommy and her baby from infancy through adulthood; *Goodnight, Moon,* a short children's classic about significant items within a home being in their proper place for bedtime; and *Put Me in the Zoo,* one of Dr. Seuss' edited books featuring an animal who keeps being told he cannot be in the zoo like he wants to be. *Love You Forever* and *Put Me in the Zoo* especially resonated with her. Bethany explained that the message of secure love in *Love You Forever* particularly meant a lot to her; she also really liked *Put Me in the Zoo* because, "It means, like, you can't tell me what to do, except if it's my mom telling me to clean up" (personal communication, December 19, 2015).

Her initial reluctance to talk with me quickly dissipated and she shared that she does not like going to the hospital because she does not know what is going to happen: "I don't know if I'm going to like be okay after" (Bethany, personal communication, December 19, 2015). While I lacked the greater context of her full medical journey, it was easy for me to see that she had been through many unpleasant and undesired medical experiences. Her discussion of her favorite stories highlighted the importance of her family's presence and support while she remains hesitant to comply with anyone or any situation that brings discomfort or pain; she has been and remains in search of control over what happens to her.

Bethany's health began to deteriorate at six years of age. Her mother, Paula, became concerned when Bethany's urine contained a high concentration of blood. After a short stay at the Stollery Children's Hospital in downtown Edmonton, it was determined that Bethany had developed post-infectious glomerulonephritis, an illness that can follow a strep infection.

Medication resolved the concerns. Soon after, however, Bethany began projectile vomiting. Following a few episodes and trips to the pediatrician's office, the pediatrician noticed some movement behind one of her eyes and that her balance was off. The doctor sent Bethany and her mother to get a CT scan of Bethany's brain; after the scan was complete, they were told to go home and that they would receive a phone call with results within a week.

Paula remembers just barely getting home from that particular visit and receiving a phone call: "They said no, come back to the hospital, she needs an MRI. And before her MRI, they told us she had a brain tumor" (personal communication, December 19, 2015). The family was devastated. Bethany was diagnosed with a Grade-1 pilocytic astrocytoma brain tumor requiring surgical removal. At the time, Paula and George did not share the results and the reality of the situation with Bethany. They did not tell her she had a brain tumor. "One of my favorite lines is 'we take care of the problems while they're small before they turn into big problems'" (Paula, personal communication, December 19, 2015). In fact, it was not until after her care was complete that her parents mentioned that she had had a brain tumor. While Bethany did not fully understand the heaviness of her situation and what was happening, she developed a matter-of-fact mind-set regarding her care. "I don't really ask questions because then I get upset and I cry. So, I kind of just let it happen" (Bethany, personal communication, December 19, 2015).

Bethany's neurosurgery was successful yet extensive, taking nine-and-a-half hours. The tumor had many fingers sitting on the brain requiring a lot of scraping in order to completely remove it. Unfortunately, the surgery came at a cost for which they were not prepared. Bethany developed posterior process syndrome causing her to lose motor function including the ability to talk and some more innate functions like keeping the tongue away from the throat in order to breathe while sleeping. She essentially was in a waking coma for nearly two months.

The fear of the unknown gripped Paula and George. Sigmund Freud (1920) suggested that fear stems from knowledge and the feeling of an inability to control the situation. Paula said, "Nobody [told] us about posterior process syndrome. That was, wow! We were just worried about [the surgeons saving] her life. We weren't even thinking about what it was going to be like [after the surgery]" (personal communication, December 19, 2015). She further expressed how they still have had to rationalize the difficult reality they dealt following her surgery:

> If you leave it—a tumor behind—it can grow up in non-operable spots, and then you're dealt with (the horrific reality of a terminal diagnosis). And also the kids would stroke out. So then [the surgeon's] finding that, yes, he's getting more kids with posterior process syndrome—nowhere near to the extent like Bethany, but he had two others that were close—but the kids have survived. (personal communication, December 19, 2015)

The months that followed Bethany's neurosurgery were incredibly difficult. George, Bethany's father, said early on that he looked at her and saw no signs of life. "Thank God the neuro-pathways started to rewire, right. But you'd look in her eyes and you'd see nothing" (George, personal communication, December 19, 2015). Bethany was in the Pediatric Intensive Care Unit

(PICU) for one week and then moved to a room in the Intermediate Care Unit (ICE) for another week. On Christmas day that year, Bethany moved to a regular room where she would stay for a little more than a month before being medically transported to a rehabilitation hospital where she would live for nearly four more months before going home on the weekends and then returning during the week for the still very needed rehabilitation therapies. In all, Bethany and her parents' lives revolved around life in a hospital setting for more than six months.

"It's just one foot in front of the other and you're just living right there in the moment because it's so intense that you can't handle anything but that moment, right. And that's what it was like for us" (Paula, personal communication, December 19, 2015). George added, "Because you don't know what you're going to end up with" (personal communication, December 19, 2015). It was that uncertainty that overwhelmed those six months, and still does to a certain extent today. Attempts to understand and cope through the present are natural techniques to manage fear and pain (Melamed, Dearborn, & Hermecz, 1983; Melamed, Meyer, Gee, & Soule, 1976; Mahajan et al., 1998; King et al., 2001; Cohen, Bernard, Greco, & McClellan, 2002; Langer, Chen, & Luhmann, 2005; Field, 2006). There were no guarantees, especially given the great extent of Bethany's presentation of symptoms associated with her posterior process syndrome. "There was the fear of the unknown. Where are we going to be in two years, in three years, in five years?" (George, personal communication, December 19, 2015).

One of the most difficult aspects of navigating the outcome of her neurosurgery was the inability to gather information and understand what was going on in order to explain it to other people. Others found it hard to listen; Frank (1995) suggested this is because "chaos" narratives are unresolved and therefore uncomfortable. Most of Bethany's caretakers did not understand her syndrome. Paula and George did receive some information from the Brain Tumor Society, but it was very limited and did not encompass the extent of Bethany's situation. As Bethany slowly recovered, she went through every development stage a second time but continually struggled emotionally. One of the rehabilitation hospital psychologists offered antipsychotic drugs but due to the lack of understanding of posterior process syndrome, it was a drug that could hurt Bethany's brain from recovering; Paula and George's instinct to question the side-effects of the drug saved Bethany. It was frustrating for them that they could not fully trust the medical professionals.

Bethany had to relearn every motor function; however, for the most part, she has. At the time of the interview, Paula reported that she is above average in her academics and has regained her ability to talk and walk. In an emotional and social sense, Bethany has caught up to her peers, as well.

While she enjoys school and playing with her friends, she must go at her own pace. Bethany deals with brain fatigue. Situations can become too overwhelming and draining. In order for her to make it through a school day, she requires naps to allow her brain to rest. In restaurants, the background noise can become too much requiring her to remove herself from the stimulation. Additionally, Bethany still struggles with handwriting and speech.

Bethany has also had MRIs, a sleep study, and an eye surgery to further follow and correct issues resulting from the neurosurgery and posterior process syndrome. The psychological and emotional trauma is still very present. Anytime anesthesia is involved, Bethany has struggled. Paula recalled how 'she did say, "I don't like being put to sleep because I feel like I'm never going to wake up." So, to me, that was, "Alright, so what does she remember [from the] long period of time that she was not [responsive due to the posterior process syndrome]?"' (Paula, personal communication, December 19, 2015). George concurred and added, "She's starting to grasp the magnitude a little. I would say probably as years go on, she'll start to realize how close [she was to death]" (personal communication, December 19, 2015).

To help Bethany with the emotional trauma, Paula explained that they take Bethany to therapy through a company, called Brain Works, which specializes in educating children about and helping them through emotional experiences. Paula even has benefited from the service. "We even sometimes go twice a week, and honestly, I credit [the therapist] a lot because she helped me deal with it. It [gave] me and Bethany so much ability to control—tricks and triggers and what to do and how to express yourself" (Paula, personal communication, December 19, 2015).

The therapist has since helped Bethany emotionally prepare for medical procedures. At the time of the interview, it had only been a few weeks since Bethany had an eye surgery to correct strabismus. Paula knew she could not inform Bethany of the surgery alone; she needed support: "Sometimes I feel like I just want to cry with her. So, I have that great support system for her; they can step in and put the [right] words" (personal communication, December 19, 2015).

The therapist put the information in narrative form; videos and pictures helped Bethany better understand what would happen. For the sleep study that happened 18 months prior and was just as emotionally traumatic as the recent eye surgery, Bethany created visual lists of comfort items to bring, which included her favorite stuffed animal and blanket, snacks, and photos. It was her first time sleeping overnight in the hospital since her six-month stay. She made a stress jar filled with water, glitter, and small sequins and foam pieces that can be shaken and watched as the glitter and small pieces float back to the bottom; it helped calm her.

In addition to their therapist and certain medical professionals, Paula and George have enjoyed attending Brain Works conferences. The resources and knowledge they have gained have helped them learn how to better advocate for Bethany. "Being educated, that really helps. It really helps when you feel like you understand what's going on" (Paula, personal communication, December 19, 2015). The ability to grasp the situation from a holistic point of view has been crucial to helping Bethany understand and navigate her experiences as they come. In many ways, this included finding ways to meet her information needs, which were often best met in visual and narrative forms.

Frankie

I met Frankie and her family the day after her thirteenth birthday. She loves anything and everything Gap. While initially unsure of whether I was truly just a visitor [and not a medical provider of some kind who might inflict some sort of discomfort], she quickly warmed up and wanted me to meet her life-size teddy bear named Ethan. Frankie is very motherly, as she made sure Ethan was not awakened while meeting me; the mannerisms she displayed while holding the bear were mind-blowing. Frankie had clearly paid close attention to how nurses and therapists care for their patients.

She also showed me her new Gap beanie and scarf full of pink, blue, yellow, and white stripes that she got for her birthday. She modeled them for me. Her attention eventually turned to Freddie, her "Elf on a Shelf" who was perched above the front door. Marta, her mother, explained that Freddie cannot be touched until Christmas Eve when Frankie can hug him before he flies back to the North Pole. She reluctantly complies. It was clear that Frankie has strong connections with people and things that hold meaning to her.

With the sun now beginning to set in the late afternoon, I sat on the comfy shaggy white rug spread across the family's beautiful dark living room wooden floor. With the fireplace keeping the home very comfortable compared to the wintry temperatures outside, Marta began explaining Frankie's medical journey. As we talked Frankie brought the family's newest member in to meet me. Miss Pip, their five-month-old chocolate labradoodle, recently joined their family as a therapy dog for Frankie. Marta said the results of Pip's presence have been amazing, and formal training has not even started.

Frankie was born with cleft lip-palate anomalies that were not detected until birth. While Marta was pregnant with Frankie there was some concern about one of the chambers of Frankie's heart, but an ultrasound at 21 weeks ruled that out. However, by the time that Frankie was three-weeks-old, Marta and her husband, Simon, could see that their daughter's health was deteriorating rapidly. After persistence on Frankie's parents' part and multiple trips to their local hospital's emergency room, it became clear that she, in fact, did have cardiac issues. An x-ray revealed an enlarged heart and Frankie was rushed to the Stollery Children's Hospital in downtown Edmonton where more tests began. At that time, three holes in her heart were found and doctors deemed it a miracle that she was even alive. Within a week, Frankie would have her first open-heart surgery.

Since then she has had many other surgeries spread out over the years. In total, there have been two additional open-heart surgeries, four surgeries to address the cleft lip and palate anomalies, a G-tube placement surgery, and a gallbladder removal surgery. Just a week before my interview with Frankie, she had a dental surgery. Additional surgeries are planned to address ongoing concerns with her heart and craniofacial anomalies.

While Frankie has had to deal with multiple operating room experiences and various hospital clinic visits, she also has had communication hurdles to overcome. From a clinical perspective, she is considered to be nonverbal with a severe global delay; she has some vocal cord paralysis, as well. However, at the time of the interview, her vocabulary and ability to speak was growing. Between her augmented tablet device, her ability to draw and gesture, and the vocabulary she does have, she is generally able to make herself understood, especially to those who know her best.

The most difficult part of her medical journey has been maintaining the medical team seeing Frankie as a whole person. Her team is comprised of 13 specialists who are mindful of their role but often forget how their piece affects the whole "puzzle" of Frankie's care. Additionally, Marta shared that, "Getting around the cognitive delay and people understanding how important it is that she is part of her care" is challenging (personal communication, December 19, 2015). This aspect of her medical experiences has greatly affected Frankie's ability to navigate through her journey of procedures.

As I was talking with Frankie and Marta, they told me about the traumatic anesthesia experience Frankie had just had with her dental surgery the week prior. Upon them arriving at the hospital, Frankie asked for an IV induction of anesthesia instead of the typical procedure of using a mask. Despite knowing that it can be difficult to get an IV going on Frankie, Marta decided to follow Frankie's lead and at least give it a try. After multiple unsuccessful pokes and Frankie in great distress with six adults holding her down, the anesthesiologist refused to let Marta hold Frankie. She tried, but they pushed her off. She suggested the mask but was ignored. Then, the anesthesiologist matter-of-factly decided they needed to move on to the mask and do so quickly. Marta described Frankie as tremoring on the operating room table—as if she was having a seizure. The anesthesiologist came up from behind Frankie's head, pushed her head down, and applied the mask.

As Marta told me this, Frankie said, "Crying. I hated it" (personal communication, December 19, 2015). The horrifically fearful look on Frankie's face as she fell asleep was still engraved in Marta's memory. In that moment, all Marta could do was get as close as possible to Frankie's face and reassure her. With Frankie asleep, Marta walked out of the operating room devastated. As she reflected back on the experience the emotions were still raw. "There comes a point where the child's pride is completely taken away. I don't care what situation happened, that should always be protected. . . . I think giving processing time for a patient like Frankie and allowing her to have more control [would have made a difference]" (Marta, personal communication, December 19, 2015).

Frankie's story was a perfect example of the importance of including children in their care. Regardless of verbal ability, Frankie's keen sense of awareness of her surroundings only reinforced the importance of involving her in the process of care and allowing her time to make sense of what was happening and how it was being done. The retelling of Frankie's story and her interjections affirm the power of narratives and the greater, collective understandings that can come from them (Japp, Harter, & Beck, 2005).

Hannah

Six-year-old Hannah was still recovering from a surgery that happened the week prior when I visited her family's home. Her beautiful silky dark hair was pulled back into two ponytails with pink and white Hello Kitty bows atop her head. She was dressed in all pink and greeted me with a smile. Hannah and her mother, Cara, welcomed me into their home. Hannah's room was just off the home's entryway; it was decorated in soft pinks and purples perfectly fitting for a precious little girl. Her room also had a shelf with a small set of drawers set up with all the medical equipment and supplies needed to accommodate her care. They invited me in to sit on the loveseat in the corner as Hannah climbed back under her blanket on her bed and Cara sat next to her.

Hannah has a tracheostomy (trache) because her tongue rolls back due to a small jaw not supporting it, which ultimately occludes her airway; she was able to talk, though, because she used a speaking valve with her trache. The decision to put in the trache was not an easy one for Hannah's parents. Cara recalled leaving the NICU (neonatal intensive care unit) around midnight one night shortly after Hannah was born only to wake up at 4 am sensing something was wrong. She called the hospital and learned that Hannah had gone into cardiac arrest because of her airway occluding. The cardiac arrests happened another eight times; while fighting back tears, Cara told me that it became clear the trache was necessary but that it was hard to convince her husband because he had a really hard time accepting the idea.

Additionally, Hannah has microtia atresia, the absence of her outer ears and ear canals, a cleft palate, along with other craniofacial anomalies. Each of the craniofacial anomalies is tied to her Treacher Collins syndrome. As we began talking, Cara explained that Hannah's most recent surgery was to do the final phase of her BAHA (bone-anchored hearing aid) implant and that she was not recovering as easily as usual. The surgery was successful, but Hannah was running a slight fever and struggling with abdominal pain in the days that followed. She cuddled under her blanket while we talked but quickly perked up when I asked her to draw me a picture of her in the hospital. Hannah loves drawing; it was a great distraction from her discomfort at the moment.

Hannah was fully aware of her medical situation and beginning to navigate the reality of others' reactions to her appearance. She has asked why other children laugh at her. When Hannah, along with her three older siblings, played at the park, Cara took the opportunity to gather a whole group of children who were laughing and not speaking kindly and to share with them how everyone was made differently. Cara tried to use it as a teaching moment for the other children and her own, especially Hannah. "I think she learns just from hearing me talk" (Cara, personal communication, December 20, 2015).

One of the most difficult aspects of navigating Hannah's medical journey was the lack of knowledge regarding Hannah's diagnosis and what other children with her syndrome typically have experienced. At the time of our meeting, they had only recently learned of and connected with two other families living nearby who also had children with Treacher Collins syndrome. Outside of social media, there was very little community with which they can connect on similar experiences.

While Hannah has had multiple operations, she has remained compliant and trusting of her parents. Cara shared that Hannah does not ask many questions; Hannah simply has relied on the information Cara has given her. Cara has found that Hannah feeds off of her emotional state; if Cara is calm, Hannah does much better throughout the entire procedure. Hannah told me, "I'm a little bit scared, [but] just talking about it and counting [while falling asleep under anesthesia helps me calm down]" (personal communication, December 20, 2015). The loving and trusting relationship between Hannah and her parents was foundational to Hannah's ability to make sense of her medical journey. This co-construction affords the needed space for reflection and interpretation in order to pursue sense-making (Beck, 2005).

Jacob

Anxious anticipation of what the next uncomfortable medical procedure might be was a constant struggle for three-and-a-half-year-old Jacob. Such a fear is one of the most common childhood phobias (King et al., 2001). Even my evening arrival at six o'clock created apprehension. His mom, Carol, told him I was just a friend coming to talk, but he had to be coaxed into waving hello upon my walking in the door. Jacob observed my every move as I took off my snow-covered boots and began taking out my recorder and papers for the interviews.

It was below zero degrees Fahrenheit that evening; roughly six inches of fresh powder covered the residential streets, which were in much need of plowing. My front-wheel drive rental car got stuck in the snow a few houses down. After maneuvering just enough to get traction, I was able to park in the family's driveway and march my way through the snow up to the front door.

Despite his being shy and unsure of my intentions, Jacob sat in his overstuffed chair in the family's living room with the most well-behaved manners; he worked on his wooden-shape puzzle and looked through his *Sesame Street* books without a fuss. Carol and I sat down opposite him so she could observe his breathing while we began talking. Jacob's trache required regular suctioning; along with the scarring from so many intubations required as an infant, bronchomalacia, weak bronchial walls, and his left vocal cord paralysis made it impossible for him to breathe without the trache. Jacob communicated through sign language; he was also learning how to use an augmentative and alternative communication (AAC) device.

Carol and her husband of six years learned of Jacob's fragile medical state while she was pregnant. Around 19 weeks' gestation, an initial ultrasound detected cardiac defects, which were confirmed and more clearly defined upon extra scans around 26 weeks' gestation. They also learned that Jacob was missing half of his cerebellum, called cerebellar hypoplasia, at 30 weeks' gestation. "There were a lot of tears and a lot of hard nights" (Carol, personal communication, December 18, 2015). It was during this time that they began to organize and construct their narrative—something that can have a healing effect (Coulehan, 1991). Carol was glad she had the time to prepare; she asked a lot of questions of her obstetrician and researched a lot online.

Time also presented challenges, though. A lot of the information she found about Jacob's cerebellar hypoplasia pertained to cats. Such little information only complicated Carol's efforts to make meaning of an already-difficult situation (Kalitzkus & Matthiessen, 2009). While it was frustrating, the lack of information forced her to put aside the task of researching online and focus on tasks that would more positively affect their situation—like establishing the foundation for what would become their story.

Once Jacob was born, the procedures began. By the time he was six weeks old, he had already undergone three surgeries, one of which was open-heart surgery. Around one month old, the neurosurgery team at the Stollery was able to avoid placing a shunt for Jacob's hydrocephalus, which was tied to his brain's anomalies, and perform a reservoir instead. The reservoir technique, if effective, treats the issue of edema and a lack of proper cerebral spinal fluid flow without introducing a foreign apparatus and catheter within the ventricles of the brain, which is known to need revisions over the course of the person's life. In Jacob's case, the reservoir has been successful.

Jacob also had a G-tube placed for feeding. He will likely have airway reconstructive surgery once the doctors are able to get his sleep apnea under control. However, the most pressing issue is addressing his torticollis, muscle stiffening on the right side of his neck causing his head to tilt slightly. Carol explained that the discussion centered on whether or not to surgically sever the muscle in order to allow Jacob's neck to stretch out and his head to straighten; the risk in this surgery was that the location of the trache was too close and his airway could be compromised in recovery.

Carol stated, "We're a long way away from yearly doctor visits and only seeing one doctor. He's got something medical happening to him very often. So, even if it's a good month and the worst thing that we do is a trache change; the trache changes are still traumatic" (personal communication, December 18, 2015). Older children who are able to communicate what a trache change feels like have told Carol that it is not painful; however, they said that the time while the trache is out feels like a pillow is being held over their face and their oxygen is cut off. The routine medical care and discomfort have put Jacob in a place where he is tired of it all, regardless of him knowing no other way of life.

Carol brought Jacob over to the couch where we had been sitting and talking. He showed me his device and used it to say, "Hi, my name is Jacob. I am three-years-old" (personal communication, December 18, 2015). As I asked him about going to the doctor, he quickly signed "all done." Carol explained that "all done" is commonly used. It is clear, though, that he finds solace in children's television shows and movies. Jacob primarily watches them on his iPad. He told me about his current favorite, Disney's *Brave,* a movie about a young princess who has resolved to live life by her own rules, and saved her kingdom from a curse through bravery and her archery skills. He also really enjoyed Nickelodeon's *Bubble Guppies' "Call a Clambulance"* episode, a cartoon story in which one of the characters, Avi, broke his tail and the doctors helped him get better; in fact, it was the one show that he routinely returned to after traumatic medical experiences.

For example, just one month prior to my visit Jacob was hospitalized for five days while he received an antibiotic infusion for parainfluenza. Carol told me how the stay was relatively uneventful; he was in isolation, had some IV starts and blood draws in addition to an echocardiogram while Child Life specialists, hospital employees specifically trained in providing emotional support for children and their families, distracted him. The events were not outside his procedural norms, but anxiety was high nonetheless. "It's the [hospital] room; he knows things are going to happen. It's everything and nothing" (Carol, personal communication, December 18, 2015). Following his discharge, Carol explained how Jacob watched the *Bubble Guppies* "*Call a Clambulance*" episode multiple times; she believes it is the reassuring message that help is coming that makes it so attractive to Jacob.

Weeks later, Jacob was still talking about that hospitalization. Each trip to a clinic for a doctor visit brings anxiety and fear that he might have to be admitted again. While his parents tried to reassure him, Jacob just wanted to leave. He had a similar reaction when he realized his trache was about to be changed. Because the changes were done at his preschool, the medical team, and his teachers implemented a visual schedule or a pictorial outline of steps to help him understand what was about to happen.

Jacob's anxiety over trache changes, various procedures, and hospitalizations were his current biggest challenges. However, the visuals made a positive difference in his ability to stay calm. Even at Jacob's young age of three, he was already seeking strategies by which to restore consonance to his situation.

Nadia

A school bus, with seven-year-old Nadia on board, pulled up in front of the family's home as Nicole, Nadia's adoptive mother, and I were talking. Nicole quickly threw on her winter coat and walked out to the curb to help Nadia off the bus. Nadia entered the front door with a smile and a Doc McStuffins themed backpack, a product tied to the popular *Disney Junior* series, *Doc McStuffins*, that shows a young girl pretending to be a doctor and treating her toys in her backyard playhouse turned clinic. She said hello to me as Nicole introduced us. While Nadia sat on the entryway floor taking off her boots, jacket, and snow pants, she quickly requested a glass of chocolate milk reminding Nicole that it was promised earlier that morning. After finishing her chocolate milk and snacks, she brought down her Doc McStuffins' play set to show me. When I asked her what Doc McStuffins does, Nadia told me, "She helps me feel better. I like Doc McStuffins" (personal communication, December 16, 2015).

When Nadia's family was preparing to adopt her from China, they were planning for palliative care. The few documents that had been released regarding the background of the then-five-year-old Nadia stated she had multiple brain tumors. However, it was the kind gesture of a Stollery neurosurgeon that would give hopeful information to Nicole, Nadia's adoptive mother.

Around two months prior to the finalization of Nadia's adoption, Nicole was at the Stollery with Peter, her adoptive son (another participant whose story is described below); Peter was seeing his speech pathologist that day when the neurosurgeon passed through a nearby hallway. Seeing the neurosurgeon, the speech pathologist asked if he would not mind taking a quick glance at a CT scan Nicole had recently received. The neurosurgeon stated that the scan did not seem to show a terminal situation but that more testing would be needed. "So we didn't know what; we just knew we weren't going to be burying her" (Nicole, personal communication, December 16, 2015).

Nicole and her husband, Timothy, first learned about Nadia from a family friend who had visited the Chinese orphanage where Nadia was living; the friend was pursuing a separate adoption but was drawn to the very shy and withdrawn girl and began advocating for her adoption upon returning to Canada. Nicole and Timothy's hearts were touched. Nicole told me that she remembers praying that God would send her a child that no one else wanted. Initially, there was a lot of interest from other families but as it dwindled, Nicole explained they pursued a medical expedite and within a few months Nicole was traveling to China to bring Nadia home.

Within a month of Nadia's arrival, she had an MRI. The neurosurgeon who initially looked at the CT scan saw Nadia in clinic and reviewed the MRI; he diagnosed Nadia with frontal lobe hydrocephalus and missing a portion of her right frontal lobe. The good news was that she did not need a shunt. The brain anomalies were due to a stroke Nadia had while she was in utero. The neurosurgeon continued to follow Nadia, especially looking for signs of cerebral palsy because it is common in children with the same anatomical presentations. Her family watched for seizures and headaches, but at the time of the interview she was stable.

Nadia also had development delays including cognitive and motor function. With underdeveloped hips, doctors were watching her development and could eventually suggest surgical treatment. Yet, in the two years since Nadia was adopted, Nicole had seen so much growth. "She really has blossomed, and I keep thinking, well, her language has come along amazingly, considering. I think she's doing very well" (Nicole, personal communication, December 16, 2015). Nadia was in a mild cognitive delay special education class that used a lot of visuals to reinforce schedules and assist in the teaching of new concepts.

Nicole recognized that the adoption process put a different spin on the information-gathering process. She and her husband wanted to know as much as they could about her medical status prior to bringing her home, but clear diagnoses had to wait until she could be seen at the Stollery. As Nicole learned more, she found the Internet helpful for further research, but she felt comfortable with what the doctors shared with her.

The language barrier and Nadia's limited emotions, due to the brain anomalies and neglect while in the orphanage, presented their own challenges for helping Nadia through scans and doctor appointments. She was very aware of discomfort and procedures that were painful. Nadia usually showed her emotions as either extremely happy or extremely sad; there was no middle ground. "I'm scared of the doctor. I cry. I cry a lot, a lot, a lot" (Nadia, personal communication, December 16, 2015).

Initially, Nicole would tell Nadia, "Butang, butang," which means "no hurt" in Mandarin, but with the growth in Nadia's English Nicole was able to explain more. Nicole explained that visuals encouraging calmness and bravery had not been used in the hospital setting but that they should have been as they would likely reduce some of Nadia's stress, especially because her school used a lot of visuals in their teaching. She further stated that doctors' use of visuals would be an added help: "[Doctors] need to learn how to better explain to those kids. Because most kids with cognitive disabilities have other health concerns, [I wish] they would be better taught or have the desire to use pictures" (Nicole, personal communication, December 16, 2015). Nadia's story pointed toward the rhetorical power of visual narratives that can help children better understand the process of their procedures and the impact they will have on the children's lives.

Nathan

Nathan, 13 years old, is Nicole and Timothy's biological son. He was their first window into the world of raising a child with special needs. The narrative processing of thoughts and emotions related to Nathan's care would only expand as additional children with medical needs joined their family; their family story would not only include the sharing of experience but also reflecting on what they had already overcome. Nathan was born legally blind, but they would eventually learn that it was delayed brain development. Today, Nathan is able to see with a little help from a pair of glasses.

Nathan had already arrived home from school when I pulled up. There was one more day of school before the winter holiday break. Upon walking in the family's home, the home's warmth welcomed me in from the brisk afternoon air. Nicole made me a cup of herbal tea and we began talking in their front room.

Nathan came to see who was sitting on the couch near his mom. He noticed my recorders sitting between Nicole and I and became curious; he wanted to touch the buttons. I explained that they record our voices and showed him the audio waveforms changing as I spoke. Nathan is nonverbal but made barking noises to see the effect. Nicole mimicked him and asked, "Are you a puppy?" (personal communication, December 16, 2015). He smiled.

At the time, Nathan had been seizure-free for 15 months with the assistance of anti-seizure medication. Outside of regular doctor appointments, his last major procedure was an MRI around the time of his last seizure. Prior to that MRI, though, his life was filled with scans, electroencephalograms (EEGs), and tests.

The clinics' waiting rooms presented the most stress for Nathan. "He used to have tons of meltdowns in the waiting room because it was so stressful for him to be in there with the noise. And I'm stressed; we're both stressed" (Nicole, personal communication, December 16, 2015). Nathan would typically calm down from reassurance and simple explanations once he was in a private room, but if needles were involved, the anxiety escalated. Sometimes visuals were used, as well. "The simple explanations are okay, but I think pictures with a social story are much better" (Nicole, personal communication, December 16, 2015). Nathan relied on patterns and routine. The visual structure helped reinforce a sense of security.

The doctors have never been able to figure out his diagnosis. "We've had every testing for developmental delay. No diagnosis, and he's had lots of testing done. That used to be kind of important" (Nicole, personal communication, December, 16, 2015). Over time, Nicole has accepted not knowing the diagnosis, especially the "why" behind Nathan's cognitive delay. "It's not the end of the world. It's tough sometimes but you'll be happy. You'll enjoy life, and you'll know who your real friends are" (Nicole, personal communication, December 16, 2015). While medical information lacked, Nicole was able to make meaning of her family's medical story through experiential knowledge (Kalitzkus & Matthiessen, 2009).

Like many of the children, predictability was crucial for Nathan. His anxiety lessened with a simple explanation of what to expect. In spite of a cognitive delay, Nathan could make sense of what made a situation secure. His story shows that the identification of information needs and the proper use of information sources are invaluable to his ability to navigate his medical experiences.

Peter

Peter, five years old, is the youngest sibling to Nathan and Nadia. He, too, was adopted from China like Nadia; they were not biologically related, though. His parents, Nicole and Timothy, adopted him nearly four years ago when he was 18 months old—two years before Nadia joined the family to make it eight strong.

Along with Nadia, Nathan, and Peter, Nicole, and Timothy have three biological daughters: Kyla, 18, Angelica, 16, and Alyssa, 9. Nicole joked, "Because it's a competition I want to win; I want those kids, too!" (personal communication, December 16, 2015). Nicole and Timothy, a Lutheran pastor, had big hearts and a desire to help others in need. Additionally, both, Nicole and Timothy, grew up with the familiarity of adoption; they both had adopted siblings. Adopting seemed natural for their family, as well.

Like Nadia, Peter took the bus home from school. He was in an early education class that included other children with speech delays. Peter was born with a cleft lip and palate. His lip was repaired in China before being adopted but his palate was not. He still had some speech issues, but they greatly improved with his last surgery that was just one month prior. As I spoke with him, he was quick to show off his new ability to articulate specific sounds. Nicole asked him, "Do you like that you can make more sounds and everyone can understand you better?" (personal communication, December 16, 2015). Peter replied with an emphatic, "Sssssss-ink!" (personal communication, December 16, 2015). He would need additional palate reconstructive surgeries to finish closing the opening in his palate.

The anxiety around these surgeries was very high for Peter, though. He understood that the surgeries helped him but that they were very painful. This reality made it difficult for Nicole to help him navigate his experience. "I don't feel like always talking to him really helps with the anxiety because his procedures are painful. He misbehaves; he acts up" (Nicole, personal communication, December 16, 2015).

The family had one picture of Peter as an infant with the cleft lip; they have shown it to him to help him see and better understand the progress he was making because of the surgeries. In the past, the surgeon also drew pictures for Peter so he could better understand the procedures. Nicole believed the visual aspect of the photo, and drawings helped Peter construct a reassuring understanding of his journey.

Just before his last surgery, he received a doll from the Stollery. The Child Life specialist brought it to him and used it with role-play to explain the process of preparing for surgery and then recovery afterward. "He got to draw the face on it. He put the numbing cream on the doll; he gave the doll the IV. So that was a huge help; I thought that made a big difference [in lessening his anxiety in both before and after surgery]" (Nicole, personal communication, December 16, 2015). It was as if the doll provided an unconventional means by which understanding could be created and a small part of his story could be shared (Kalitzkus & Matthiessen, 2009).

In the meantime, Peter not only continued to receive speech therapy within his school, but he visited the Stollery's speech clinic every couple of weeks, as well. Besides the cleft lip and palate, his family kept tabs on his nephrodic syndrome, a kidney disease that causes severe fluid retention. Peter was hospitalized for it six months prior to the interview. Nicole explained that Peter should outgrow the syndrome.

Throughout the four years since bringing Peter home, Nicole felt very prepared and that her information needs were met. In fact, she had an appointment scheduled with a plastic surgeon from the cleft lip and palate clinic before she ever left for China to bring Peter home. The online support communities for adoptions with cleft lip and palate also offered a plethora of coping tips and a huge emotional support. In addition to the increased ability to communicate as Peter's English improved, the advantages of more information and resources, in comparison to the lack of information and preparation for Nadia or Nathan's diagnoses, indirectly benefited Peter and his family's ability to help him navigate his medical experiences.

Taylor

Taylor and her mother, Amy, were unavailable to meet while I was in Alberta, so we arranged to speak over FaceTime during the afternoon of New Year's Eve before, ironically enough, the Edmonton Oilers and Anaheim Ducks would face off that night. You see, Taylor and her family traditionally cheered on the local Oilers; I shared that my favorite team was the Ducks.

She was a fairly shy twelve-year-old girl but Taylor warmed up to me pretty quickly and we struck up a fun conversation. Amy and Taylor sat at their kitchen table while I found a quiet corner in the timeshare my large family had reserved for the week. As we began talking, I realized Taylor was born with a very similar craniofacial condition as my daughter, Reagan. We had a lot in common, which made for a very easy conversation and interview despite it being over FaceTime.

Taylor's official diagnosis is a syndromic version of craniosynostosis causing the plates of her skull to fuse early in utero; this further made for limited room for other anatomical growth within her head. "Everything kind of went where it had room to grow. So the result of that is her ear canals, her eye sockets—the holes in her head for a lack of a better term—are pretty small for what they need to do" (Amy, personal communication, December 31, 2015). Taylor's first surgery was a craniotomy at nine months of age and helped to open up and correctly shape the skull.

When she was three years old, Taylor had another surgery to open up her eye sockets and make her forehead a bit stronger. She needed additional surgery to enlarge the pathway that her right eye's optic nerve traveled; the optic nerve was being pinched. The surgery was not successful, though; the optic nerve could not be saved causing her to lose vision in her right eye.

Taylor has also had her adenoids removed, multiple MRIs, and sleep studies. Sleep apnea is very common in children born with craniosynostosis; to help Taylor with this, she uses a C-Pap machine each night. At the time of the interview, Taylor had recently received the diagnosis of scoliosis, which is related to her Jackson-Weiss syndrome. However, the neurosurgeon was hesitant to allow surgery to correct the scoliosis because of Taylor's chiari malformation, which happens when a portion of the cerebellum is lower than it should be and can extend into the foramen magnum and possibly involve the brain stem. In the meantime, Taylor wore a back brace to help with the scoliosis. She was also anticipating a mid-face advancement surgery at some point, a surgery known to have a difficult recovery. "That's not anything we're rushing into" (Amy, personal communication, December 31, 2015).

Taylor has always had an easy-going temperament. Amy explained that even when she woke up from her surgery at age three with an eye sutured shut, "She just kind of rolled with it; she kind of just accepts situations that she's been in and makes the best of them" (personal communication, December 31, 2015). Taylor told me she remembered feeling alone when lying on her bed before going under anesthesia, but she tried to stay calm. "I just knew my parents told me that I'd be safe—like I'm fine—and that I would be okay" (Taylor, personal communication, December 31, 2015). She also kept one of her Stuffie stuffed animals nearby for comfort. In moments of pain and difficult recovery, Amy and Taylor usually snuggled, sang, and read stories. When Taylor was younger, she loved reading *Little Quacker,* but there was nothing significant about it; it was more of an activity that allowed them to be together.

The relationship Taylor shared with her parents fostered a sense of security regardless of the fearful procedure or difficult recovery. "We would just talk about it in terms that we could all relate to; she's always understood that all of the things we're doing is to just help make her a strong, healthy person" (Amy, personal communication, December 31, 2015). It was in this narrative construction that they each found a place to articulate, reflect, and listen (Frank, 1995). The trust Taylor placed in the information her parents shared with her played a significant role in her ability to navigate her medical journey. They, as a family, have learned to appreciate the little things and not be afraid to advocate for Taylor's best interest, which included seeking answers and information as they were needed.

SOUTHERN CALIFORNIA INTERVIEWS

Throughout my journey with my daughter, I, too, have had to learn the importance of asking questions, advocating for my child, and organizing our story in such a way to best encourage patient-provider communication that allowed her to remain fully human (Frank, 2001). Part of this growth has come in seeking out various activities that might have some therapeutic value and possibly meet a need of my daughter. Because of it, I have crossed paths with various medical professionals and other "medical mamas" who helped me gain access to the following families. Each family lived in the general Southern California area making it easy for me to travel to interview them in person.

Brooks

I met 12-year-old Brooks and his mother, Linda, at a Coffee Bean coffee shop. We all grabbed a drink and a breakfast pastry before heading outside where it was a bit quieter and easier to talk. There was a nice spacious area with almost 10 or so tables spread across the patio that separated the coffee shop's doors and the parking lot. The weekend morning air was a bit brisk, but the skies were clear after an overnight rain. The chairs showed signs of the rainfall. Linda chose a table near a planter in the middle of the patio and after wiping off the chairs we sat and began talking.

Brooks was a bit shy and tired. Initially, he lowered his head and allowed his mom to talk with me. Linda explained that her 12-year-old son catches up on his sleep during the weekends. During the week, the family schedule requires him to wake up around 5:30am to get to school.

He was born with microtia artesia, a craniofacial anomaly that happens when one or both ears do not fully form. For Brooks, only his right ear was affected. In addition to the lack of a typical outer ear, he did not have an inner ear canal or the ability to hear out of that ear. When he was six years old he had the first stage of plastic surgery to remove the unformed portion of the ear and attach a new fully formed aesthetic ear made of a polyethylene material that was compatible with living tissue and modeled after his parents' ears. Just a few months prior to the interview he had a second surgery for minor revisions on his ear. Brooks also had oral surgery due to the right side of his jaw not growing proportionately.

For Brooks, the surgeries were about self-confidence. He did not remember being bullied or made fun of, but he did have the desire to appear like his peers. "If people see the ear, they don't say anything because it looks like the real ear" (Brooks, personal communication, January 10, 2016). Linda was always aware of this aspect of her son's social life; even as a single mother, she made the sacrifice to keep her children at the same school with the same group of friends regardless of moving to a new city or job.

The choice for going forward with the surgeries was always Brooks' decision. The concern about how the final product would look and if it would hurt was at the forefront of his thoughts. These concerns were met by information provided in videos. His plastic surgeon produced videos with photos of the surgery to give patients and families simple step-by-step explanations of what would take place. The videos were designed with the use of very clean images, but those that Brooks saw as a five-year-old boy still remain in his memory seven years later.

Brooks drew a picture of him getting ready for his surgery; he was alone with the anesthesiologist receiving his IV in preparation for the surgery. Nervousness and a desire to have the surgery behind him consumed his thoughts. Brooks told me that he imagined that the children in his plastic surgeon's videos also felt similar: "[They were] scared or just wanting it to get over with and not knowing what is going to happen next" (personal communication, January 10, 2016).

Linda sat across the table watching and listening to Brooks as he described his picture. She was shocked at his feelings of being alone. "[Parents] say something different, [like] 'I love you,' but did they hear? No, they don't hear. Or [parents say,] 'I'm here for you,' but the picture [that Brooks drew says,] 'I'm alone.'" (Linda, personal communication, January 10, 2016) Linda explained that she believed Brooks imagines the situation more how the videos portrayed the situation; no parents were shown in them. She is saddened by the impact the videos had on Brooks. "It's the picture you have, and you can have it all your life. It's no way to have a happier life" (Linda, personal communication, January 10, 2016).

Brooks' experience affirmed the use of media with medical themes to explain medical procedures and help children make sense of the situation. Such mediated stories are successful because they reference the defining human activity of narrative construction (Bruner, 1986). While the context and surrounding activities of the procedures must also be considered, they allowed for basic information to be shared, understood, and experienced. Brooks and Linda suggested that the inclusion of parents in the videos explaining the ear reconstruction surgery would have benefited Brooks and provided him with a more reassuring remembrance of the experience.

Kyler

A televised National Football League game could be heard from outside Kyler's home when I knocked on their front door. It was Sunday afternoon and playoff football had arrived. Jenna, Kyler's mom, opened the door and welcomed me in; Chris, Kyler's father, greeted me, as well. Jenna and Chris have two boys. Kyler had turned eight years old two months prior. He and his two-year-old younger brother played very well together in the hallway off the living room despite their age difference.

Kyler was born with bilateral microtia artresia; both of his ears were underdeveloped at birth. At the time, the family was living in San Antonio, Texas. The appearance was not a concern for his parents; however, the hospital staff could not initially explain what had happened to his ears. That immediately started Jenna and Chris on a path of seeking meaning for what would become their story. They asked a lot of questions and looked for answers. There was one nurse that first night who directed them toward a plastic surgeon who performed aesthetic ear reconstructive surgery. After talking with that doctor, they pursued placing Kyler in a special Parent-Infant Program at a deaf school that encouraged the use of hearing aids; this allowed them to hear others' stories. The co-construction of their experience as they walked similar journeys with other families led them to a knowledge of Cochlear, a hearing aid implant company, and helped them begin to make sense of circumstances that resisted sense-making at the most fundamental of levels (Beck, 2005).

As parents, their support network grew. They had heard many families' stories regarding ear reconstruction making them comfortable about presenting it as an option to Kyler. "We met one young girl who had her surgery, and he just looked at the ears and said, 'Oh, okay!'—like [it's] just a typical kid" (Jenna, personal communication, January 10, 2016). They also showed him photos and videos of other children who had had the surgery. "I think seeing [that] another kid [with] the same condition, and [she] went through the surgery and look at her, she's fine. So I guess the before and the after was okay; [as if Kyler would say,] 'she's okay so I'll be okay'" (Jenna, personal communication, January 10, 2016).

Prior to his surgery, the family had attended a convention in San Diego sponsored by Cochlear. At this conference, Kyler received a stuffed moose named Vibe (for vibration) that also had BAHAs in his head. Vibe also came with a coloring book that told the story of his BAHA implants. Kyler became attached to the stuffed moose and took him into the operating room on the day of his surgery.

He had his first aesthetic ear reconstructive surgery a month before his birthday while he was still seven years old. While the surgery can be performed as early as three years old, Jenna and Chris wanted to be sure that Kyler truly desired the surgery for himself. It was about a year prior to the surgery that he decided he wanted ears like his parents. At the time of the interview, the right ear was healing very nicely and the left ear was scheduled for reconstruction in about six months. Kyler proudly told me that the best part was: "I got big ears now; I'm like everyone else" (personal communication, January 10, 2016).

The excitement and optimism overshadowed any doubts Kyler had going into surgery. He told me that he was, "A little bit nervous and scared a little bit [about] if I could feel anything" (Kyler, personal communication, January 10, 2016). With one ear reconstruction behind him, Kyler's biggest mental obstacle is trusting that the ear is strong enough to withstand sports. The surgeon approved him to play; Kyler had to learn to trust that his ear can take the contact.

Kyler's medical journey displayed how important it can be for children to play a role in their medical care. The use of visual and narrative means to share information with Kyler had a significant impact. With the information shared in a positive manner, he was able to construct an understanding that provided a sense of security.

Leslie

I first met Leslie and her mother, Kim, at a local community dance class for preschoolers. Kim placed Leslie in the class with the hope of further encouraging balance, coordination, and flexibility. Leslie was almost three years old at the time and had been recently diagnosed with cerebral palsy as a result of medical malpractice at the time of her birth.

While Leslie was a baby Kim noticed Leslie staring and making strange arm movements while laying in her crib. Suspicious that they might be seizures, Kim began video recording them. One night when she was 14 months old the "episodes" continued to happen; Kim took Leslie to the emergency room, and after doctors looked at the video, Leslie was admitted to the neurology floor under a preliminary diagnosis of seizures. While in the hospital multiple EEGs were done but none showed the same activity that was happening at home. However, the doctors did order a lumbar puncture; that revealed the cerebral palsy. At this point, different specialists who saw Leslie disagreed regarding the movement being related to her cerebral palsy or whether it was specifically tied to seizures. The decision was made to put her on seizure medications, but after a couple years, Kim and her husband felt it was best to wean her off of them due to the negative side-effects of the drug. At the time of the interview, Leslie had been seizure-free without the medication.

Leslie was also followed by an orthopedist for the curvature of her pinkie fingers that related to the cerebral palsy. The curvature is progressing causing peers to take notice. "She was crying about it to me one night because she felt that she was being made fun of for that. So, I explained to her that she was born that way [and to tell her classmates that she likes the way she was born]" (Kim, personal communication, January 10, 2016).

Since her cerebral palsy diagnosis, however, Leslie has had multiple EEGs; the last one was about a year prior to the interview. As Kim and I sat in her family room with faint sounds of Leslie and her daddy playing together upstairs in the home's loft, she explained that familiarity and repetition have not lessened Leslie's fear surrounding the EEGs. "It was still very hard on Leslie because she was older and she absolutely hated it and thought it was the worst thing in the world. We had a really hard time explaining to her why she was going in" (Kim, personal communication, January 10, 2016).

Leslie used to love Disney Junior's *Doc McStuffins,* the television series that showed a young girl treating her toys in her backyard playhouse; Kim stated that they used it a lot to help demystify visits to the doctor, but that she had outgrown it. However, Leslie was becoming very interested in science; she regularly watched YouTube videos about the human body and played apps that had medical content designed for children. Leslie also liked

Disney's *Pirates of the Caribbean*; they referenced the movie when Leslie needed x-rays. "She likes skeletons, and so [I said to her], 'Really! Oh, you want to see pictures of your bones?' She just thinks they're the coolest things" (Kim, personal communication, January 10, 2016). Other stories allowed Leslie to co-construct her own health story.

The goal was to minimize Leslie's anxiety by explaining procedures in a way that she could make sense of the information in as concrete of a way as possible. This included simplifying information as best as they could and using visual and narrative forms, specifically media that had medical ties. While some of the media were not created to be medical information sources, the family was creative to maximize the resources available to them and use that which connected with Leslie.

Reagan

Reagan's story was first introduced in the Introduction. Since that described hospital stay, she has had multiple surgeries including a shunt placement, a laminectomy to remove spinal cord cysts, two eyelid ptosis repairs, and numerous sedated MRIs. In addition to these procedures, she has continued to see multiple specialists including a neurosurgeon and plastic surgeon.

She was diagnosed with bicoronal craniosynostosis within days of her birth. As her team of specialists grew, Reagan began seeing a geneticist who identified a displaced anus requiring pediatric surgery at five months of age. A month later Reagan had her major craniotomy to initially correct her craniosynostosis. While she was in the PICU, her geneticist informed us that her craniofacial anomalies were in fact related to a syndrome. Additionally, she had other genetic deletions that were unnamed with unknown risks. The best the geneticist could tell us was to remain vigilant regarding all major organ functions.

At thirteen months, Reagan was beginning to crawl well. Her gross and fine motor development were delayed. However, she began experiencing extreme neck pain. After multiple admissions and tests, her neurosurgeon diagnosed Reagan with a spinal cord syrinx that would eventually require a chiari malformation reconstruction surgery at three years of age.

That surgery did not heal well and within six weeks she had contracted bacterial meningitis requiring a 21-day-long IV antibiotic treatment and the shunt placement. As a result of meningitis, Reagan developed spinal cord cysts. Those cysts caused her to lose almost all desire to eat, have extreme headaches, and to feel very nauseous and light headed. The laminectomy removed most of the cysts; some whose removal could cause permanent damage were left. Reagan continued to have routine MRIs to check on the status of her shunt and the cysts. As she has grown, plastic surgeries were also required out of medical necessity.

The most challenging aspect of her medical care was managing her anxiety, especially just prior to a procedure when a team of multiple doctors and nurses work around her. "When I see people, I scream. Because people are around me; I just want it to be us" (Reagan, personal communication, January 20, 2016). Reagan deeply relied on those with whom she felt safest.

As mentioned in the Introduction, the desire to find ways to help Reagan take ownership and thereby better navigate her medical experiences had become a deep passion of mine. She always enjoyed books. At the time, one of her current favorites was The Berenstain Bears' *Hospital Friends* books, which pleasantly introduces children to the happenings within a hospital. Reagan was quick to point out that the entire Berenstain Bears' family is in it; the representation of reliable relationships is important to her in the midst of so much instability. I would be remiss to not also note the impact that media with medical themes has had on Reagan's ability to make sense of her medical journey. So much of her understanding about procedures came through relating her experiences to those of characters she had seen in cartoons and storybooks like *Doc McStuffins*, *Bubble Guppies,* or even the personal narrative featuring her favorite stuffed lion, Brave Dave, which I put together in a digital story form on her iPad. She often referred back to the connections she had made with these characters and the points of security in spite of such uncertainty that were indirectly communicated.

Victor

The El Nino rainstorm that Southern California was anticipating hit the night before my interview with three-year-old Victor and his mother, Cindy. That morning as I pulled up in front of their apartment, I realized I forgot my umbrella. I parked as close as I could and ran to escape the pouring rain. A very happy Victor greeted me once his mom opened the door. Despite his limited vocabulary, it was clear that Victor wanted to play cars with me. "He loves cars. Cars are his favorite. If this child is able to, I am going to tell you right now, he's going to be a NASCAR driver" (Cindy, personal communication, January 5, 2016).

Victor was born with a severe cleft lip and palate. He also received diagnoses including deviated nasal septum, autism, cerebral dysfunction, developmental delay, hearing impaired, sleep apnea, and muscular weakness. As Cindy and I began talking she explained that Victor was still recovering from his latest cleft lip and palate surgery—his fifteenth surgery and nineteenth time to go under anesthesia overall. This recovery was going more smoothly than others; he was eating, and Cindy was grateful for that.

In telling their story, Cindy has learned to reflect on and cherish the small triumphs. At 26 weeks' gestation, the doctors found Victor's cleft lip via ultrasound. Victor was also measuring small for his gestation age. Cindy remembers being encouraged to do an amniocentesis and then being offered abortion. "I told my husband, 'No one is taking my child but God. I'm not doing [the amniocentesis] and I do not want anyone to offer me termination again.' So, I signed all that paperwork and then went home and cried" (Cindy, personal communication, January 5, 2016).

Her emotions fueled her desire to be as knowledgeable as possible. She set out on a quest to face the diagnoses and allow their story to become one of overcoming (Frank, 1995). However, in this effort to satisfy her need for information, she created more fear for herself. Cindy explained, "I Googled to my own detriment. It's hard. I was afraid that I was going to be scared of my child when he was born because, I mean, the pictures they have online are obviously like the more severe" (personal communication, January 5, 2016). As she prepared for his birth, she focused on loving him for just how God created him: "He was beautiful just as he was. What was I so scared of?" (Cindy, personal communication, January 5, 2016).

At four months of age, Victor had his first surgery to place ear tubes in an effort to release fluid buildup and increase his hearing. Then at seven months of age, he had his first lip repair. Before Victor turned one year old, he would have a G-tube placed and another lip repair surgery. At the time of the interview, he had had six surgeries related to his cleft lip and palate alone.

The rate of therapies and doctor appointments per week were high, as well. Since Victor was a baby they have had at least one appointment per week, and Cindy told me they currently average around three appointments with as many as seven or eight in one week. "This is our life. This is our world. There's no different. This is normal to us" (Cindy, personal communication, January 5, 2016).

Despite the routine nature of therapies, doctor visits, and even surgeries, the anxiety of painful procedures caused Victor to shut down when they arrived at the clinic or hospital. "He stops talking completely. There's no babbling or anything. He just stares. He won't walk; I have to carry him" (Cindy, personal communication, January 5, 2016).

In preparation for procedures, Cindy explained that she tries to talk to him using words he can understand while they are still at home; she also, when applicable, shows him pictures from past procedures. For the last surgery, Victor understood that he was going to have a "boo-boo." "I think he gets some of it; I think he gets enough of it" (Cindy, personal communication, January 5, 2016). However, it remained hard for Cindy to see him cry and beg for no boo-boos. Although she stated that he had improved; he used to scream, especially if there was an unfamiliar experience.

While we played cars and colored together, Victor repeatedly told me, "Later at the doctor I get boo-boos. No, not today" (personal communication,

January 5, 2016). It was as if he was reassuring himself. His concept of doctors had not reached an appreciation for the work they've done to help him come as far as he had; he associated them with pain.

Victor's information needs remained simple. He needed to know if there would be pain and what exactly would be done. The family struggled, however, to find information sources to best meet his needs. In spite of this, Victor remained resilient, a testimony to the supportive relationships that surround and nurture him.

Wyatt

Four-year-old Wyatt attended preschool with my twins, Rhyan and Jordan. Wyatt and Jordan, both, love Transformers: Rescue Bots. When I arrived at Wyatt's home around dinnertime on a Thursday evening, he showed me the Rescue Bots he had and asked which ones Jordan owned. Wyatt was comfortable with me because he had seen me many times before around his school.

With Christmas just a few weeks away, Wyatt told me all about the toys he wanted to get as presents. From his living room couch, we looked out the window at all the Christmas lights and decorations spread across his family's front lawn. It really was a beautiful display. He was a happy boy.

Roxanne, Wyatt's mother, sat nearby and tried to eat her dinner while she had a few free minutes. However, Wyatt's baby sister woke up and wanted to be held. Roxanne explained that the two are polar opposites when it comes to sleep. Wyatt's often excessively tired while his little sister struggles with sleep.

Wyatt was born with spina bifida requiring a spinal closure at two days old. Because he also had hydrocephalus, he had a shunt placed at six months of age. Wyatt also had a chiari malformation, which was finally addressed at age two. "His entire brain stem was being smashed, so they were able to relieve the pressure" (Roxanne, personal communication, December 10, 2015). He since has had a shunt revision, which helped alleviate some of the sleepiness.

Navigating Wyatt's medical journey has been hard for Roxanne and her husband. They felt their chaos story, as Frank (1995) would put it, was difficult for others to listen to and understand—even by medical professionals. Wyatt's medical issues were complex, and his care was often incomplete. "I had to do a lot of research myself and kind of look into things. . . . If it wasn't, again, for more research, I wouldn't have known to go back to our doctor. And a lot of times, especially depending on your insurance, the doctors are sent so many patients and they're just looking for the bare minimum, and you kind of have to be your own advocate" (Roxanne, personal communication, December 19, 2015).

In spite of the tough journey, Wyatt has been resilient. Wyatt uses braces to help him walk. However, he cannot run. Roxanne explained, "We'll go to parties and he can't run or ride a skateboard or the bike, and so he'll just go play by himself. I don't think any of that's going to register until he probably gets a little older, but I think to him everything is normal" (personal communication, December 10, 2015). She added that Wyatt has not asked why things are different, but that she has tried to help him understand why he needs the medical care.

Roxanne has used the simplest terms as possible in preparing Wyatt for an upcoming procedure, like an MRI. "He doesn't like it, but I just tell him, 'Hey, we're taking a picture of your head to make sure it's okay'" (Roxanne, personal communication, December 10, 2015). Wyatt's anxiety drastically increased when the medical staff would not allow Roxanne to be with him during an MRI while she was still pregnant with Wyatt's younger sister. Roxanne pleaded her case that she had been in a four-hour MRI while pregnant with Wyatt, but the staff did not budge. Instead, they had to restrain him, and he screamed for the entire MRI. Because of that experience, every MRI since was called the "noisy bed." "Now he won't cooperate at all. He used to cooperate" (Roxanne, personal communication, December 10, 2015).

Wyatt overheard his mom talking about the "noisy bed." He came over to us. I asked Wyatt if he liked the MRI and he answered, "No, because it makes noise. BAHHHP . . . BAHHHP . . . BAHHHP" (personal communication, December 10, 2015). When I asked him what he thought of doctors and nurses he told me that they call him for the MRI and because of that he does not like them.

It is very frustrating for Roxanne. Distraction no longer works. Instead, Wyatt fixates on his anxiety and whatever procedure about which he is upset. Even after it is over, he repeatedly talks about how much he hated it. In those instances, Roxanne has tried to reassure him: "I remind him again when he complains about his head or his back (that) we're just trying to check it and make sure everything's okay. (I) just kind of leave it at that; there's not much (more to say). I just let him vent and just go from there" (personal communication, December 10, 2015).

In those difficult moments of Wyatt's anxiety, Roxanne's role has had to become focused on just getting him through the situation rather than finding ways to help him navigate the situation with understanding. She wished doctors and nurses would, "Be more understanding of why the kid's fearful or upset. It almost seems like they're so busy that they don't take the time to make sure they're comfortable or they're okay" (Roxanne, personal communication, December 10, 2015). Wyatt's story showed how important the use of rhetorical information sources can be. In the moment of procedures, Wyatt's anxiety was too high to recall the simple conversations he and his mom had had.

Part of navigating children's medical experiences is for parents, caretakers, and medical professionals to have the tools to meet them where they are at and help them make sense of what is happening and why. These health narratives show that making-sense is possible, although it may come by means that are not yet considered conventional. The long-term impact of medical experiences on each child's life has begun to be revealed. As we move forward, there is greater understanding as specific lessons are exposed.

Chapter 2

Making Sense of the Difficult

The complexity of these children's challenging medical journeys has the potential to influence their worldviews while shaping their character and the people they are becoming. Children who spend a lot of time in the hospital with frequent medical procedures live on the margins of life. Their experiences are the vulnerable antithesis of the hopes and dreams epitomized in the idea of a young child (Eilertsen et al., 2009).

People make sense of their experiences differently, yet they share common routines making for collective outcomes. They frame their experiences to make sense of situations while maintaining a positive self-conception (Goffman, 1967). Brown, Stacey, and Nandhakumar (2008) noted that while "much sense is shared, [people] are strategically motivated to determine their own highly personal interpretations of what has occurred" (p. 1052). Brown et al. (2008) posited that narratives are indeed persuasive in how meanings are understood, ultimately affirming that sense-making of individual micro-level stories helps to make sense of organizational macro-level stories. For these children, situations are often framed in some sort of a unique rhetorical manner. To add to this, family members must also facilitate their own sense-making experiences to not neglect but rather maximize their well-being (Davidson, 2010). This can be difficult as parents must find ways to make sense of the situation and navigate through fearful experiences while also assisting their child in the same process.

These children and their families navigate fear, the potential of social rejection, pain, and uncertainty on a regular basis. To most their experiences are foreign, but to them their journeys are their "normal." In spite of the great lengths that parents and medical providers go in order to create a comfortable and kid-friendly environment (e.g., bright colors and creative designs that make the hospital feel less sterile), the children have a heightened sense of awareness regarding their surroundings and who is present. An individualized approach is necessary.

Gillis (1990) supports the notion that, when possible, preparing children for medical procedures and hospitalizations is helpful in reducing anxiety. However, a difficulty of preparation efforts is that younger children struggle to verbalize their hospital-related fears outside of the hospital environment (Broome, 1986). In fact, Broome (1986) found that very young children are "more situation specific in their fears than are late school-aged children" (p. 144). Attempts to prepare young children should not be completely abandoned, though. "Very young children can provide important insights into their health experiences, so their views can and ought to be taken seriously" (Salmela, Salantera, Ruotsalainen, & Aronen, 2010, p. 113).

For Bethany, her drawing's detail (e.g., the interior decorating, equipment, and even the entertainment set-up) was meant to distract her from focusing on the discomfort of the situation depicted; this shows just how much of an impact the totality of an experience can have on a child (see Appendix B, Bethany). She mentioned her disdain for the presence of the sleep study technician and drew him very small in comparison to her; this revealed the desire to push him out of the situation. Bethany also drew tears and a screaming thought bubble showing the intense emotions that the situation produced within her. Attempts to fool these children and mask the inevitable discomfort are nearly futile.

Hannah's drawing (see Appendix B, Hannah) of the anesthesiologist preparing her trache for surgery also supports these children's keen awareness and the memorable impact of their experiences. As Hannah drew, she explained her intentional choices of color. Cara, her mother, affirmed her memories of how the hospital gown was green, the anesthesiologist's scrubs were blue, and how the anesthesiologist had some facial hair and wore a head wrap along with brown boots. Hannah explained that she did not like the anesthesiology experience, but she trusted the doctors and nurses. Her extremely detailed memory, which included specific articles of clothing and their colors, shows just how aware these children are during each procedure.

Patients need the security of knowing that they will have the help and information they need to survive whatever procedures come their way (Waska, 2012). A child's ability to make sense of situations requires guidance (Zangori & Forbes, 2013). This sense-making process can entail multiple techniques and can come from multiple information sources that ultimately lead to children's heightened engagement in learning and exploration (Alfieri, Brooks, Aldrich, & Tenenbaum, 2011; Honomichl & Chen, 2012). Children place their trust for information to aid in the sense-making process in the adults overseeing their medical care. The trust placed in parents, caretakers, and medical providers is grounded in a need for feelings of security

(Giddens, 1991; Ladd, 1992) and largely based on perceived competence and having good intentions (Ahmad, Ferlie, & Atun, 2013). Additionally, Erickson, Sroufe, and Egeland (1985) noted that a child's relationship, beginning in infancy, with the primary caregiver lays the foundation for the child's social-emotional development. A secure attachment with meaningful adults positively affects the child's confidence and ability to navigate through difficult situations (Erickson, Sroufe, & Egeland, 1985; Bowlby, 1982).

As information sources are accessed and children begin to construct an understanding of their situation, sense is made and anxiety is reduced (Fernandes, Arriaga, & Esteves, 2014). The cultivation of information through various sources helps prepare a child for what may lie ahead within their medical journey (Jaaniste, Hayes, & von Baeyer, 2007). Children's sense-making is rooted in this ability to prepare and have a perspective offering them reproducible behaviors that encourage hope despite their difficulties.

TOO MUCH OF THE FAMILIAR IS STILL TOO MUCH

Throughout the interviews the children and their families repeatedly noted a distinct understanding that their experiences were unique to those with complex medical diagnoses. For many of the children there was no other known reality, and yet they resisted the difficult experiences as if they knew life should not have to embrace such anxiety and pain. For example, Carol explained, "[Jacob] is just hyper-aware of everything to do with medical-anything. He sees a stethoscope, and he is concerned. Blood pressure assessments in-home have him asking if we are going to have to go back to the hospital" (personal communication, December 18, 2015).

Prior experiences further impact children's life perceptions and the lens by which they view the future (Jaaniste et al., 2007; Klingman, Melamed, Cuthbert, & Hermecz, 1984; Melamed et al., 1983; Melamed et al., 1976). Marta, Frankie's mother, told me a story of when Frankie had seizure-like behaviors inside a store at their local shopping mall. At the time of the interview it had been four years since the episode and four years since Frankie had been back to that store. Just two weeks before I met Frankie, she and Marta walked past the store in the mall; Frankie recognized it and acted out the experience: "She pointed at the store and [shook] her whole body. We've never talked about it; it just blew my mind" (personal communication, December 19, 2015).

It is this degree of memory that points to children's deep awareness of their medical journeys. Marta added that it was because of this awareness that care must be taken to protect future experiences. While discussing the difficulty of getting Frankie into the operating room for her most recent surgery, she stated, "I know that wasn't her last time, so how does this set her up for the next time?" (Marta, personal communication, December 19, 2015). One experience impacts how the journey ahead will be navigated.

The anxiety experienced in the past can even spill into environments that are designed to provide comfort. For Victor his home is a safe space, but our discussion about his last cleft lip and palate surgery triggered concern over whether his environment would have to soon change and he would be experiencing a painful procedure that day. When I asked him about his recent "boo-boo," Victor adamantly stated but with slight inquisition, "Not today. No, maybe I get a boo-boo on my nose. No, later" (personal communication, January 5, 2016). He was processing through the familiar possibility of leaving his home for the hospital.

Pain, uncertainty, and loneliness are just a few of the recurring emotions that accompany these children's awareness of the difficulty through which they must process during their medical journeys. With each new procedure, their heightened awareness of the difficulty is affirmed (Fernandes et al., 2014). While Victor and I talked and he drew a picture of himself in the hospital (see Appendix B, Victor), he was sure to draw the doctor last and far away after he first drew his mother near him; he also resisted simply drawing anything more than a dot for the doctor. He told me, "I don't like it!" (personal communication, January 5, 2016). In fact many of the children stated that very same thing.

Reagan, who has had more than 30 experiences of anesthesia in her six years of life, holds a strong aversion to "falling asleep" for a procedure or surgery. "I don't like the stinky mask. It's stinky. It's scary" (Reagan, personal communication, January 20, 2016). Her experiences point to the significance of finer details that give greater meaning to the larger context. When talking with Reagan she spoke of her dislike for the tape that is used to affix IVs, bandages, and other medical materials. She also specifically mentioned the way unfamiliar people make her feel: "When I see people, I scream because people are around me. I just want it to be us (i.e., her, her daddy, and me, her mommy)" (Reagan, personal communication, January 20, 2016). Reagan's drawing (see Appendix B, Reagan) focused on the moment her MRI was over; she drew herself with happy anticipation for the rewards she was promised upon the completion of her MRI. When asked why Reagan did not want to draw any of the difficult aspects, she emphatically explained that she did not like them.

Bethany similarly pointed out specific characteristics of her hospital experiences including her dislike of the presence of the medical team. "I don't—to be honest—I don't really like to be in the hospital because it's like everyone's staring at you and like watching your every move" (Bethany, personal communication, December 19, 2015). As previously mentioned, even when Bethany drew her picture, she resisted and drew the technician very small showing her dislike for him. For children who journey through complex medical situations, the intended communication of care through a medical professional's watching over a patient can be misinterpreted and further complicate the children's experiences.

Sometimes small individual difficulties become too much to bear. "It is nothing and everything because the nurses were nice; he wasn't left alone. He had an IV start. He had a blood draw, which is traumatic, but he'd had those before. . . . It's the rooms that he knows [are places where] things are going to happen. It's everything and nothing" (Carol, personal communication, December 18, 2015).

SUPPORT STILL DISAPPOINTS

For these children, somewhere between everything and nothing lie the painful procedures that contribute to the difficulty. While drawing a picture of him at the hospital, Peter began with him lying on a gurney. He next drew an IV tube attached to a pole that stood next to him. Peter told me he was crying in the picture. What happened next though was very telling; Peter pressed into the table with his crayon and scribbled out the picture he had just drawn (see Appendix B, Peter). When I asked why he colored over it, he said, "Because I like to" (Peter, personal communication, December 17, 2015). He then explained that when he was in the hospital he just wanted to go home. While he did not articulate the initial impact of the pain from the needle poke, in addition to the pain of his surgical recovery, the intentional coloring over his picture showed his desire to remove the pain altogether. "(Peter) understands that his surgeries are painful. [A cleft lip and palate] does hurt and it's quite a painful surgery for them" (Nicole, personal communication, December 17, 2015).

There is little reprieve from the pain. For Bethany the familiarity with certain procedures did not lessen the frustration that accompanied her pain. As we talked, she told me about her recent eye surgery and her latest sleep study—both of which held memories of discomfort. The sleep study, which she chose to draw (see Appendix B, Bethany), required the placement of electrodes all over her head, which were applied with a sticky paste that pulled on her hair when removed; an IV was also placed. Through the night as she tried to sleep, the technician came in her room to adjust the electrodes. She told me she screamed inside her head. Bethany also explained how she has had multiple IVs since her initial cancer diagnosis five years prior; however, the nurses' repeated attempts to get a good vein in preparation for her last eye surgery were almost more than she could bear: "The second one and the third one feels like crushing your brains" (Bethany, personal communication, December 19, 2015).

Of the 11 children who had the ability to draw, nine children (i.e., Bethany, Brooks, Frankie, Hannah, Kyler, Leslie, Peter, Taylor, and Victor) depicted scenes that involved some element of physical discomfort or pain. Seven drew needles and IVs. Of these children, five (i.e., Bethany, Brooks, Kyler, Leslie, and Peter) drew blatantly sad expressions with Bethany, Brooks, Leslie, and Peter also specifically drawing tears (see Appendix B).

Through the pain, the children recognized the support of family, but the harsh reality was that it disappoints; it could not take away the pain. Just a few days prior to my interview with Leslie, she had been to her orthopedist after breaking her arm. The team attempted to reset the broken bone but could not do so due to the extreme pain it was causing Leslie. While this procedure was unrelated to her more complex medical diagnoses, it was traumatic nonetheless. As Leslie drew the doctor attempting to reset her arm (see Appendix B, Leslie), she told me it hurt but that her mom tried to comfort her. "She was trying; she was right next to me, but I kept on crying and it kept on hurting" (Leslie, personal communication, January 10, 2016). Leslie ended up needing anesthesia in order to properly reset her arm. The pain, coupled with the lacking ability to engage in other routine activities due to her broken arm, had profound impact on Leslie's capability to handle the procedures involved: "No one understands how a physical injury can set your child back. She's not able to really play, . . . so she's not getting any sensory input or release" (Kim, personal communication, January 10, 2016).

As children attempt to make sense of their stories, isolated medical experiences must be attended to with care. While it is Kim's hope that Leslie is able to one day recall positive aspects of her journey as she reflects back, there is an undeniable struggle to acknowledge and attend to the suffering. Perhaps it will be the strategies created with the intent on helping children navigate medical fears and pain that influence children's development and impact their well-being later in life (Salmela et al, 2010).

THE JOURNEY IS STILL EVER UNPREDICTABLE AND LONELY

Uncertainty is manifested in a child's lack of security regarding how a procedure will feel and what a situation's outcome will be. The fear of pain itself compounds the difficulties a child faces throughout a medical journey (Kennedy et al., 2011). Additionally, anxiety stems from a child's inability to confidently predict what will happen next (Jaaniste et al., 2007). For example, Wyatt's anxiety over the uncertainty of pain and when he would be separated from his mother further compounded the difficulty of his MRI experience. Hannah, too, shared about the uncertainty surrounding her surgeries in spite of her familiarity with the process. She explained that no amount of information brings assurance and makes her comfortable.

The navigation of uncertainty also includes the determination of whether a procedure would or would not bring discomfort. As Kyler drew a picture of himself in the operating room just before his ear reconstructive surgery (see Appendix B, Kyler), he described himself as nervous and scared. When asked why he felt that way, Kyler answered: "Just if I could feel anything" (personal communication, January 10, 2016). When I asked Brooks about his surgeries, he similarly expressed that he knew they were for his benefit, but uncertainty of the situation made him nervous: "Just if it hurts or not, . . . like if I feel like it's going to stay with me—that pain" (personal communication, January, 10, 2016).

"It's scary because I don't know what's going to happen" (Bethany, personal communication, December 19, 2015). The internal quest to predict the future for a sense of safety and rest was ongoing. Even parents struggle with it. Cara, Hannah's mother, admitted, "I don't even know what the next step is or when the next step is. . . . [The medical providers] don't even know" (personal communication, December 20, 2015). The uncertainty transcends young children's inability to understand standard protocol; when caretakers are unable to communicate some semblance of predictability, the medical journey's difficulty causes the children to turn inward.

The feeling of loneliness was a surprisingly common thread that ran through my discussions with the children, especially in light of the fact that these children's medical teams were large and each of the participants had parental support. For example, when I asked Brooks to draw a picture of him in the hospital, he drew himself receiving his IV for anesthesia just before his last ear reconstructive surgery; the drawing included only a doctor and him lying on a bed. As Brooks explained that no one else was with him, his mother, Linda, sat near him at the table and became noticeably sad for him. Linda was moved to share about her fears of being abandoned following her divorce; she likened her feelings to what Brooks drew. "I have been with him all the time before and after the surgery, but he pictures himself just with a doctor and a bed and just—it's not here how it was. . . . No support [and] abandonment; it's one of [his] fears" (Linda, personal communication, January 10, 2016).

Taylor also drew herself alone in a hospital bed with an IV, despite having space available to draw other people (see Appendix B, Taylor). She described herself to me as sad and scared when discussing her drawing. "I should have drawn my parents and the doctors, but I . . ." (Taylor, personal communication, December 31, 2015). Taylor could not finish her thought. She silently shrugged her shoulders. After a bit of silence, I asked her if she felt alone even though people surrounded her, and she sighed, "Yeah" (Taylor, personal communication, December 31, 2015).

The sense of loneliness is an expression of these children's attempts to navigate the difficulties of their medical journeys. Uncertainty and pain were prominent, as well. Throughout the data, though, the discussion of an IV was pronounced. This repeated inclusion of an IV might not simply represent a frequent occurrence for these children and a routine part of their medical procedures; rather, the IV tubing and its connection to a pole, which in many ways is stationary, may in fact hold significance to the children regarding limits they learn to live with and restrictions by which they refuse to be controlled.

YET STILL PUSHING PAST THE DIFFICULT

While the children were aware of their surroundings and realized that difficulties accompanied them on their journeys, they maintained a resiliency. This resiliency created hope in the midst of suffering and manifested itself in a physical and an emotional sense (Whiting, 2009). Children who have complex medical diagnoses carry within them an innate strength to fight against the odds. For many of the children, their lives were considered miracles. As Marta, Frankie's mother, put it: "We've come a long way!" (personal communication, December 19, 2015).

Frankie is a perfect example. Because the three holes in her heart and the interrupted aortic arch—all of which should have been operated on upon birth, went undetected and undiagnosed for the first three weeks of Frankie's life; many doctors feel she should have died. Once an x-ray revealed an enlarged heart and she was finally transferred to the Stollery Children's Hospital, Frankie's medical team warned Marta and her husband that the prognosis was not good. "At that time, they didn't think she'd make it, to be honest with you, but clearly she has" (Marta, personal communication, December 19, 2015).

The outlook on Bethany's future quality of life also was dismal for many weeks following her neurosurgery. Her medical team did not fully understand her comatose-like state. Paula, Bethany's mother, shared:

> It was them not knowing what posterior process syndrome was and not knowing how to make it better for her with her ataxia and her emotional [state]. So, when Bethany started coming back, it wasn't like we all of a sudden had a six-year old back again, right. We had an infant back. She went through every stage, from toddler to [a young child]; she learned to speak and what her emotional stuff was. And so, it was really—the hardest thing was [the] unknown. (personal communication, December 19, 2015)

Bethany remembered with pride the day her mouth began cooperating with her brain. "It was relieving because [I] finally got it. I remember this one time when my speech therapist came in and I started to sing the alphabet" (Bethany, personal communication, December 19, 2015). Before this point, she told me it had been very frustrating not being able to communicate. Through a lot of hard work, hours spent in therapy, and determination, Bethany eventually regained her other motor functions, as well. At the time of the interview, Bethany still struggled with brain fatigue but she had managed to stay on track academically. "She's above average in her class, right, even though she's missed 60% of school since Grade 1" (Paula, personal communication, December 19, 2015). Paula added that they felt very fortunate.

Reagan's inability to walk within a few short weeks following multiple neurosurgeries left her neurosurgery and physical therapy team a bit baffled. She was certainly weak, but the brain signals just did not seem to connect with her legs. There came a point when a wheelchair was being considered. Yet within just a day of making that phone call, Reagan woke up and began walking from her bed to me. We knew we were witnessing a miracle. Very few developmental milestones have come easily, but Reagan has never given up. There has never been a conversation about working hard to beat the odds or a discussion about remaining strong in spite of challenges, but Reagan continues to press on to reach goals her medical team places in front of her. She seems aware that she has to work harder and that there are differences between her and the abilities of her peers, but those differences have not tainted her drive to overcome; if anything, there has been a positive peer pressure that has helped her be resilient.

The challenges these children overcome create very meaningful realizations. These epiphanies speak volumes to a child's emotional resilience, as well. Some of the children were just beginning to articulate the impact of these insights. For others it was their parents who were in awe. This resilience is intimated in the following descriptions:

Brooks, reflecting on what he has learned through his experience with having plastic surgery on his unformed ear, said: "No matter what—if you're different or like the same as people, people will treat you how you are being. Like if you're being mean, they'll be like mean to you. Since I had the surgery, I feel more like [being] glad and being nice to others. So, when I'm nice, they know that I've been through some stuff and they want to help me" (personal communication, January 10, 2016). Brooks had learned that his actions toward others could overcome any stigma associated with his microtia atresia.

Kim, Leslie's mother, sat in awe as she realized all her daughter had overcome:

> I know that I have God, and He's shown that time and time again. . . . I don't know—like sometimes you feel like you're in the middle of an emergency and it's one emergency after another, but other times you can stop and breathe and

> you look back and you go, 'Oh my gosh! Did we really just go through all that? Did we really climb all those mountains together?' Although I should say, 'Did my daughter climb all those mountains?' because she's the one who did all that hard work and all those therapies. (personal communication, January 10, 2016)

There is an element of physical resiliency on the part of the child that leads to a contextual emotional resiliency for those intimately involved in the child's medical journey.

Amy, Taylor's mother, commented on Taylor's temperament: "She was like a four-year old—three or four-year old little girl—waking up from a surgery and wasn't able to open her eye, which was kind of unnerving. She just kind of rolled with it; she just always kind of rolls with it. She kind of just accepts situations that she's been in and makes the best of them. . . . She's been pretty easy to be in the hospital with" (personal communication, December 31, 2015). Taylor's easy-going attitude helped her recover more quickly and find her identity outside of her craniofacial anomalies.

As Hannah drew her picture (see Appendix B, Hannah), she expressed how there was little that could be done to take away her fear and make her comfortable as she prepared for surgery. In spite of this, Hannah drew the anesthesiologist and herself with smiles showing the emotional resilience that lies within her. At a young age, she is able to recognize and identify with, even if it is on a subconscious level, the belief that good can come from the pain of surgery and the hope that there is the possibility of a better situation beyond the present.

The following two comments are perhaps the most telling of these children's abilities to display emotional resiliency. At the time of my interviews with both Victor and Frankie, they each had just experienced a traumatic surgical experience. The pain and fear involved had been great but both of their mothers shared about the resilience displayed with deep pride for the character displayed in their children.

Cindy, Victor's mother, shared: "He will smile at you. He will sit there and they'll poke him eight times to get blood out of him—holding him down; there's four of us holding him down [while he is] screaming and yelling. Afterwards, he'll give [the nurse or phlebotomist] a high five—give me a high five!" (personal communication, January 5, 2016).

Marta, Frankie's mother, told me: "It's interesting because as soon as she comes out of the OR, after this type of an experience (i.e., a very traumatizing anesthesia procedure before surgery), she's always so—like she needs to hug me—and then everything's fine. So, I think she feels it just as much as I do; it's just on a different level. [It's] the same with the nursing staff, too. Anytime they do blood work or anything, as soon as they've done it, she needs to hug them" (personal communication, December 19, 2015).

Regardless of cognitive ability, being verbal or nonverbal, or any physical limitation, children who journey through countless medical experiences make sense of them by not dismissing the difficulty of their situation but rather creating a new normal through an ideological understanding of who they are. There is a clear empowering as the children look past the current pain. With the help of their families, children learn that there is hope. In spite of being very aware of the pain, uncertainty, and loneliness, these children are not constrained by the difficulty.

Chapter 3

Constructing Understanding in the Midst of the Trauma

Children rely on their parents, caretakers, and medical professionals for assistance in meeting physical and emotional needs; their informational needs are just as great, but might be often overlooked. Yet this need should not be surprising. Time and time again throughout my interviews, the parents hinted at their ability to cope with receiving disheartening diagnoses and disappointing news by seeking out information on their own; the information gathering process appeared to be therapeutic for them.

Although young children lack the ability to read medical literature and critically search the Internet for answers, their desire for a sense of security in the midst of uncertainty is ever present. They look to others to provide that security by means of the most basic of information: (1) What are the physical implications? (2) What is the process? and (3) What will the end result be?

WHAT ARE THE PHYSICAL IMPLICATIONS?

When I asked Jacob if he liked to know what procedures would happen and what they involved before they took place, he adamantly nodded and signed, "Yes" (personal communication, December 18, 2015). He is not alone. Every parent and child acknowledged the need for time to process through the medical situation, especially when the procedure involved physical discomfort.

Hannah's mom, Cara, explained what she tells Hannah when it is time for another hospital visit and surgery:

> When she was young, you'd take her in [and] even though she wasn't able to verbalize, right away there's this anxiety that's there; it's like you have to say, "It's okay," and give her a hug, right. Basically it's just reassurance and just

> talking at their level—not making it so—not lying to them really, but saying to them, "Yes, it might hurt, but they won't start until you're asleep so you won't feel it. Afterwards, when you come out of surgery, you are going to feel a little bit of pain, but we can give you some medication for it so it won't hurt so much. And then it'll go away; it will get better." (personal communication, December 20, 2015)

The fear of pain can dominate children's thinking about medical procedures and cause them to withdraw (Jaaniste et al., 2007; Kennedy et al., 2011). Bethany told me she wanted to know if a needle would poke her or if she would have to breathe through the gas mask for anesthesia, but there came a point when the details would be too much: "I get upset and I cry. So, I kind of just let it happen" (personal communication, December 19, 2015). The desire for information is very present, but knowledge is not enough.

WHAT IS THE PROCESS?

For children who live in a sense of uncertainty, there is a key need for and reliance on knowing when and how a procedure will happen. Nicole, Nathan's mother, shared how crucial it was to not only explain what would happen ahead of time but then re-explain each thing that the doctor does as it happens: "For any kid you've got to prepare, but especially for any kid [for whom] transitions are tough" (personal communication, December 17, 2015).

Understanding the process can focus on one very basic component of creating an overall sense of security. For Bethany, the idea of another surgery was upsetting, and understandably so. Even though it had been a few years, the remembrance of developing posterior process syndrome as a result of her last surgery—on top of her understanding that there would be uncomfortable physical implications while anesthesia was administered and then post-operatively as she recovered—was enough to make her resist the whole process. Paula, her mother, along with their counselor explained the process to Bethany and helped her work through her emotions. When it came time for the pre-op appointment with the anesthesiologist, Bethany told me she was most concerned with knowing how long the appointment would take. In the end, "it took like two hours waiting and then it was like a five second appointment. So it was talk, talk, talk, and done" (Bethany, personal communication, December 19, 2015). She explained the unexpected lengthy wait was annoying because she did not have a fully charged iPad tablet, and it ended up dying. Bethany's point about knowing the length of time involved is another example of how these children desire complete predictability for a semblance of security.

Just a few weeks prior to my meeting with Jacob, he had been admitted for a five-day inpatient antibiotic treatment. Carol shared that his anxiety lessened significantly once he was able to predict what would happen each day: "It's interesting, though, because he did get to a point where he knew his little routine in the hospital and in the room" (personal communication, December 18, 2015). She also pointed out that because of his lessened anxiety, the medical staff was able to get other tests and procedures done in his room that were too traumatizing in prior attempts.

At times the children's information needs about what would happen needed to be simplified. Hannah's mother, Cara, knew that Hannah was aware of the procedure and its process, but in the end she recommended a basic task, "I say, just count to 10 and it'll be done before you know it" (personal communication, December 20, 2015). When talking with Hannah, she told me she did get a little bit scared before going under anesthesia, but that talking about it and counting like her mom suggested helped.

Knowing the process can also include the steps needed to arrive at the desired result. For Kyler that meant he wanted to know how his "little ears" would become "big" like his parents. He saw photos and videos about the reconstructive surgery on the surgeon's website. The family also met with the surgeon prior to surgery: "She [i.e., the surgeon] told me that she's going to make the shape of my mom's ear" (personal communication, January 10, 2016). Jenna, Kyler's mother, told me that at the surgeon's prompting he also acknowledged that he wanted to know if the surgery would hurt. "She was like, 'No [it won't hurt]; you're going to go to sleep, and when you wake up, it's all going to be gone and be done'" (Jenna, personal communication, January 10, 2016). Children desire to know what steps will be taken to help minimize pain and discomfort.

WHAT WILL THE END RESULT BE?

Kyler's understanding of the process led him to the awareness of what his new "big ears" would look like. His parents, Chris and Jenna, were careful to give Kyler the time he needed to be sure he could comprehend the change that the surgery would bring: "It's not affecting my physical body. So, we wanted to wait a little bit later in his life [with the idea] that he can hopefully grasp more of what's going on, and he can make more of an informed decision and not just be, 'Oh well, Mom and Dad said get the surgery and I'm getting the surgery'" (Chris, personal communication, January 10, 2016).

After the time spent with the surgeon, looking at photos, and talking, Kyler decided for the surgery and when asked, "Why do you want to do it? He said, 'Well, because I want to have ears like you and Mommy'" (Chris, personal communication, January 10, 2016). Even as a young child, knowing the end result helped Kyler confidently choose to go forward with the surgery.

Brooks, who has had two ear reconstructive surgeries—one at age six and another at age 12—seemed to especially need the knowledge of what his ear would look like post-operatively prior to both surgeries: "If it's going to look good, or if it's just going to be like how I imagine it to be. Like if it's going to be looking like a real ear—just the same thing as last time" (personal communication, January 10, 2016). These children, especially those undergoing plastic surgery, must enter a very vulnerable place and surrender aspects of their appearance, a very real part of a person's identity (Tajfel, 1978; Tajfel & Turner, 1985; Hodkinson, 2002).

Cleft lip and palate children are similarly impacted. Not only are these children undergoing craniofacial plastic surgery, the majority of them will also spend countless hours working with a speech therapist perfecting sounds and velopharyngeal function. Much of Peter's treatment has included explanations of why procedures are needed. "The speech therapist explains it to him, right, in simple terms: 'You have to do this to open your palate'; he understands that. He understands part of his diagnosis is that [his speech is] hard to understand, right" (Nicole, personal communication, December 17, 2015). When talking with Peter, he proudly demonstrated his recently acquired skill of being able to say the "S" sound thanks to his most recent surgery. Nicole asked him if that made him happy and he replied with a confident, "Yeah!" (Peter, personal communication, December 17, 2015).

Children's information needs include a foundation of understanding regarding what the physical implications, the process, and the final outcome will be. This is helpful in identifying the most basic of information they are attempting to assimilate. Additionally, the construction process of such information can be most effective and more clearly understood in the context of relationship.

THE IMPACT OF RELATIONSHIP ON UNDERSTANDING AND SENSE-MAKING

It is in children's interactions with those around them and their sources of information that we learn what children's roles are in constructing an understanding. Children's relationships and how secure they feel with those directly involved in the situation also impact how the communication of the information is framed for them and who or what exactly are the information sources. As part of each family's variety of strategies for how to influence their child's construction of understanding, both active and passive approaches can be used. Regardless of which approach is deemed to work best, children deserve the opportunity to play their own unique role and not be compared to other pediatric patients.

Cindy, Victor's mother, put it this way: "He's a child with his own medical needs. Just because another child with the same thing reacts one way doesn't mean he's going to react the same way. What works for one kid doesn't work for every kid. It's okay to try what worked before, but when it doesn't work, don't force it" (personal communication, January 5, 2016).

The child's role is a necessary consideration. "[One of the biggest challenges has been] people understanding how important it is that she is part of her care" (Marta, personal communication, December 19, 2015). This is most easily recognized when children actively seek information.

Active Construction of Information

The children's desire for relationship was an incentive behind their active construction of understanding. Both, these children's parents and the children, desired to see the establishment of relationships that fostered a sense of security. This was actively accomplished when the information exchange included the child, related to something the child found meaningful, and connected with others. Leslie's mother, Kim, summarized it as being kid-friendly and suggested, "Talk to her, and don't just talk to me. I know this might sound weird, but take off your lab coat. [Leslie] would go to occupational and physical therapy . . . because I think she thinks it was something akin to a party place because it was so much fun for her and made for kids" (personal communication, January 10, 2016).

Including these children in the conversation about their care and communicating concepts in age-appropriate fashion is especially important and gives them a sense of control (Mitchell, 2012; Jaaniste et al., 2007)—something they desperately need. Amy, Taylor's mother stated, "As [Taylor] gets bigger, it's about her, right? So, she needs to know what's going on" (personal communication, December 31, 2015). Carol also explained that Jacob actively seeks information out of a need for ownership: "He needs to have control over his situation" (personal communication, December 18, 2015). Marta concurred and explained that regardless of physical or cognitive ability, these children should be included: "We've always talked with [the medical team at Frankie's] bedside. It's kind of a thing that yes, she has a severe cognitive delay, but I think she still understands a lot more than we give her credit for. . . . This kid has an amazing memory" (personal communication, December 19, 2015).

Perhaps that type of memory is because there is significant meaning associated with an idea or event. When something holds value or importance, the children are motivated to construct understanding. For five-year-old Peter, his active construction of understanding related to his cleft lip and palate surgeries consisted of a sense of security and whether specific types of comfort would be available. When I asked him what he did to not be scared in the hospital, Peter, seeking assurance, asked his mom, Nicole, if she would stay with him. I followed up by asking how it made him feel when his mom was with him. Peter stated, "Uh, they have Popsicles, and she brings them to me!" (personal communication, December 17, 2015). Nicole explained that Peter's asking for Popsicles became a routine while he was in the hospital. The Popsicle is one example of how an item of comfort can represent far more; Peter's request symbolized his seeking out of the secure and significant presence of a dear and reassuring relationship, which in his case was with Nicole, his mom.

Prior to surgery, Brooks told me he desired to know how it affected other children: "How many people have this problem, and if they have, like, been feeling bad, and just knowing what I could be feeling" (personal communication, January 10, 2016). Brooks' questions for his surgeon came in the consideration of how his situation related to others. Kyler, too, sought information and reassurance. To help Kyler better construct understanding, he and his parents, Chris and Jenna, attended a convention providing him opportunities to see and talk with other children who had had similar surgical care. "We met one young girl who had her surgery with [the same surgeon], and he kind of just looked at the ears and said, 'Oh okay. It's just a typical kid.' [After that it was like,] 'Okay, whatever'" (Jenna, personal communication, January 10, 2016).

Chris also described a time that was significantly moving for him as Kyler's father:

> I remember getting him off the truck [at school]. He's like, "Hurry, Dad! Hurry, Dad!" Like well, hurry for what? And then I noticed in the corner of my eye, there was a boy—they were pushing him—and he was in a wheelchair. And he's like, "Hurry up because my friend—I want to walk in with my friend!" I'm thinking who is his friend? I looked over there and I saw the kid in the wheelchair, but in my head, that's not his friend, right? So, when [Kyler] ran up, that's who he walked up to, and he was kind of holding the arm of the chair; he's going in with his buddy. I remember that morning—like I broke into tears—because we see children with certain conditions and sometimes tend to look away. It's just me being ignorant, [but] it was like he just taught me a lesson. (personal communication, January 10, 2016)

This incident showed how Kyler had constructed a deep understanding of acceptance regardless of body features or ability and a refusal to be constrained by them. This was actively done through relationship.

The interaction with other children who were also experiencing medical journeys of their own played a significant role in these children's construction of understanding. Nathan, for example, had found a great deal of security at school within the presence of other children who also had cognitive delay: "Now that he's with other kids at the same level, he's happy. So, I think he must understand [his medical situation] at some level" (Nicole, personal communication, December 17, 2015).

At the age of 13, Frankie, too, found considerable security as she interacted with babies and much younger children who were also in the hospital. Marta, her mom, shared with me that while some parents and children cringe when sharing a room with a baby, they are actually very grateful. "Well, for us, it was the best thing that could happen because all [Frankie] wants to do is to take care of that baby, and she recovers [so much more quickly] because she's more focused on that" (Marta, personal communication, December 19, 2015). Frankie's active engagement with another child requiring medical attention seems to indirectly provide a calming sense of understanding regarding the medical care she receives. Like Frankie, some children need information beyond the reassurance that close relationships can provide; this is when they actively seek ways to construct understanding.

Passive Construction of Understanding

If children sense a high level of security within their relationships, trust is established and displayed (Marshall, 2016; Filova & Sikorova, 2015). And in so doing, they no longer have the need to actively seek information but rather they leave that task to another person who they feel has their best interest in mind. Taylor, for example, shared how she did not ask questions because she felt secure with the medical staff taking care of her and that she trusted her parents: "I feel like I know a lot that I need to know. I do trust [the doctors and nurses], . . . and I just knew my parents told me that I'd be safe—like I'm fine—and that I would be okay" (personal communication, December 31, 2015).

This passive construction of information also shows the influence that is set by the emotional tone of those the child trusts. "[It's] as long as I'm calm about [the situation]. I find [Hannah's ability to trust] all depends on how everybody else in the environment is toward it" (Cara, personal communication, December 20, 2015). Cara explained that it was clear that Hannah did not like her surgeries or other procedures, but she understood they helped her; she never questioned why. "It really stems from myself as a mom [and] how I'm reacting to her and what she has to go through" (Cara, personal communication, December 20, 2015). When I asked Hannah about whether she is inquisitive and wants to know what the doctors will do, she replied, "I'm okay with what the doctors tell me" (personal communication, December 20, 2015). The example that Cara sets, along with the trust between her and Hannah, shows that one relationship's sense of security can also help build rapport in relationships with other caretakers.

Carol shared a similar sentiment. Specifically for her son, Jacob, who struggled with expressive language, this sense of trust transcended his closest relationships to other interactions with those who cared for him if the proper tone was set. She described this tone to be: "If it's as well-handled as possible, as calm as possible—you know, 'this is how it's going to be and everyone's doing this to make sure that you feel better' sort of thing" (Carol, personal communication, December 18, 2015).

COMMUNICATIVE FRAMING TO RESTORE CONSONANCE IN CONSTRUCTING UNDERSTANDING

At some point throughout these children's medical journeys, they have moments where all efforts to construct information are suspended. It may be due to complete trust in parents or caretakers, but it often relates to the children experiencing dissonance. While children with diagnoses requiring regular procedures acknowledge the difficulty of their medical journeys, their desire to resist and not be defined or constrained by them shows their longing for cognitive consistency.

Cognitive dissonance theory proposes that individuals seek consistency within themselves through the congruent ordering of attitudes, beliefs, and behaviors (Festinger, 1957). When there is disagreement among these, dissonance is created. In order to reduce dissonance and reestablish consonance, Festinger (1957) posited that individuals either: (1) change beliefs about the situation, (2) change actions or behaviors within the situation, or (3) change attitudes or perceptions (Festinger, 1957). Koppers and Cato (2008) expanded upon Festinger's research and found that making light of whatever is causing dissonance may be effective in restoring consonance.

Children's information-seeking dealing specifically with their medical conditions and experiences can certainly be seen as an attempt to restore consonance. These children experience dissonance when their beliefs about their situation being scary and/or painful are in direct opposition to the values held regarding how their doctors and treatments are meant to help them. An example of this dissonance is seen in Hannah's trust in the doctors but still not liking the situation and stating that nothing could make her comfortable.

Additionally, the children's resistant behaviors, such as when Frankie required multiple people to hold her down so she could undergo anesthesia or Bethany and Reagan's screaming, create dissonance as they do not correspond with the healing and helpful values placed in medical treatment. As these children construct an understanding of their situations, they are in fact adding to and changing their worldview. While the details of this change are unique to each of the children, overall they represent an attempt at reestablishing consonance and seeking inward peace that comes from making sense of their situations; this can involve putting a trust and confidence in the children's parents and caretakers, constructing an identity that places value on life in spite of difficulty, and finding hope enabling them to be resilient and restore consonance.

Comments such as these show how the children clearly desire consonance in the midst of their trauma:

- "His way of dealing with it is he just tells me he hates it. 'I hate that bed'" (Roxanne, Wyatt's mother, personal communication, December 10, 2015).
- "He doesn't resist, but he doesn't make any effort to help you. He's like, 'Fine, if we're going to do this, it's all on you'" (Cindy, Victor's mother, personal communication, January 5, 2016).
- "He doesn't want to deal with the process anymore" (Linda, Brooks' mother, personal communication, January 10, 2016).
- "'I'm just done. Just do it, and we're done.' She didn't want to do it at all. She was done with hospitals. She didn't want anything to do with it, and we'd finally go. Paula tried to talk about it, [but Bethany would say], 'Just take me there, and just do it'" (George, Bethany's father, personal communication, December 19, 2015).
- "Walking through the hospital, you could just see his anxiety building, and he kept telling me he wanted to go home, go home, go home. Then he was signing about the hospital, 'I have to stay in the hospital, and I'm not staying at the hospital.' . . . I think he's reached a point where everything's been too much" (Carol, Jacob's mother, personal communication, December 18, 2015).
- "[On why she loves the book titled *Put Me in the Zoo*] It's like you're not the boss of me, . . . [like you have to put me out;] you can't keep me in the sleep study" (Bethany, personal communication, December 19, 2015).

Other children demonstrated dissonance while drawing their pictures. Frankie, for example, refused to draw a needle or IV as part of her picture (see Appendix B, Frankie); she also did not want to draw the anesthesia mask. When I asked her about the doctor that she drew she stated, "He put the mask on me" (personal communication, December 19, 2016). She added a firm no when I asked if she liked the mask.

While Nadia attempted to draw her picture, I asked her if mommy talked to her about going to the doctor. She told me, "My mommy says—(silence and shrugs shoulders)—I don't know. . . . What's your name again?" (personal communication, December 17, 2015). She did not want to talk about or draw the doctor; she changed the subject and put down the crayons.

As Reagan began to draw, she told me she would draw herself during an MRI (see Appendix B, Reagan). However, she did not draw any aspects that usually have brought her anxiety. Instead, Reagan drew the toys she brought with her and discussed her desire to "get a muffin from the cafeteria and get a toy from the store if Mommy lets her" (personal communication, January 20, 2016). She desired to create consonance by distancing herself from the fearful and painful aspects associated with her MRIs.

Wyatt also changed the subject while we were talking about his shunt surgery. He began telling me about how he had headaches but quickly redirected the conversation's focus. We then began talking about two of his friends at preschool. In moments where dissonance was anticipated or apparent, the framing of all communication became very important.

These children were aware of the discomfort involved in their journeys, and while resilient, they still preferred to create dissonance between themselves and their procedures (Mitchell, 2012). In order to help these children create consonance and feel as secure as possible in the midst of their suffering, information seemed to be best framed in specific ways. Positivity with simplicity, honesty, and items of comfort ensured success within the children's construction of understanding.

The Hegemony of Positivity

Much of the concept of positivity is a hegemonic device that influences the entire framework of children's construction of understanding regarding their medical situations. The creation of an identity that is larger than these children's diagnoses and the procedures they face provided the foundation for how they seek information and further construct understanding. For example, Kyler had grown up with the freedom to talk about his microtia atresia. When he asked his parents why he was born with small ears, they used the opportunity to help him understand he was no different than another boy who wears glasses for poor eyesight or uses a wheelchair because his legs cannot effectively walk:

> In your case, you were born with small ears. . . . The worst thing you can do is put your head down and maybe shy away from it. So, look tall and put your chin up and say this is just how I was born. [If people] see confidence and your ability to explain what's going on, then you're going to be okay. (Chris, personal communication, January 10, 2016)

Jenna added, "We didn't use his small ears as a disability or an inability to do anything" (personal communication, January 10, 2016).

Kim, too, desired that Leslie have a positive identity, one grounded in a biblical understanding of who God made her to be. This sense of identity helped Leslie to be more compassionate toward others in spite of experiencing teasing at school. "Having cerebral palsy isn't easy, but it's kind of like what Joseph said, 'What was meant for evil God used for good.' [I tell Leslie,] 'See if you didn't have cerebral palsy, you wouldn't be able to be such a good friend to [a young family friend] who struggles to communicate'" (Kim, personal communication, January 10, 2016). Leslie's seeking of information about her needs and those of others is rooted in acceptance.

This type of positive identity is evident in each family. Life is valued and hope is maintained providing space for information to be positively shared. Even when medical findings or treatment suggestions are not ideal, the preservation of positivity allows children who cannot fully grasp the complexity of their situation to better navigate the journey. "I explain it as much as he can [understand. Wyatt] doesn't like it, but I just tell him, 'Hey, we're taking a picture of your head to make sure it's okay'" (Roxanne, personal communication, December 10, 2015). Explaining the situation in simple terms at the child's level of comprehension provides them the best opportunity for a successful construction of understanding.

Taylor's focus is on the end result. With this perspective, her parents have helped her see past the difficulty of her present situation. "All these things were a pain to go [through]—sit and wait at the doctors or have different procedures or have different things done—but she's always understood that all of the things we're doing is to just help make her a strong, healthy person" (Amy, personal communication, December 31, 2015). Taylor told me, "[My parents] make it into words that I can understand" (personal communication, December 31, 2015). She added that she feels confident about her ability to understand the procedures of her medical journey.

Perspective is the biggest key to framing information in a positive and simple fashion. For a child who is medically fragile and is far from simply having annual doctor visits, Jacob relies on knowing that relief from the discomfort of his present procedure is imminent. "I just try to relay to him that he's safe and that just wait, then we'll be done and focus on that we'll be done quickly" (Carol, personal communication, December 18, 2015). After the procedure is done, Carol mentioned that he often seeks out further reassurance.

Frankie often struggles most with understanding what has happened after the procedure is behind her. Marta shared that it is in the reviewing of what Frankie has accomplished that Frankie gains more confidence and security for the next procedure. "It's nice to be able to say, 'You've done this. You've done this. You've done this. You've done this.' You can see that she's like, 'Oh, I can see some relief in this'" (personal communication, December 19, 2015).

Hannah, too, benefits from reviewing a procedure. Cara, Hannah's mother, shared about the conversation she had with Hannah following her last surgery. She stated that it was mostly about talking at Hannah's level:

> I said, "Was that so bad?" And she goes, "No." And I said, "So, then next time if you have to have that, you wouldn't have to be so scared, right?" Talking about it afterwards [makes it so] she doesn't think in her mind that it's something really negative for the next surgery because it will happen again. (personal communication, December 20, 2015)

The Necessity for Honesty

A positive outlook about past experiences helps to position a positive maintenance of perspective regarding how the present fits into a larger context (Mitchell, 2012). This does not, however, take away from the need to be honest about the difficulty in the present. "Not lying to them, but saying to them, yes, you're going to have an IV in your hand, perhaps, and yes it might hurt, but they won't start until you're asleep so you won't feel it. [Or] when you come out of your surgery, you are going to feel a little bit of pain, but we can give you some medication for it so it won't hurt so much" (Cara, personal communication, December 20, 2015).

Wyatt has struggled with MRIs ever since he had a bad experience with a technician not allowing his mom, Roxanne, to be in the room due to her being pregnant at the time with his younger sister. "I just let him vent and go from there. [The MRI is] something that has to be done, unfortunately. [So I reassure him,] 'We're just making sure you're okay'" (Roxanne, personal communication, December 10, 2015). Roxanne's affording of time for Wyatt to process through his frustration and anxiety while maintaining an honest but positive stance about the need for the procedure and why it's beneficial helped Wyatt feel heard; consequently, he was better able to accept the situation.

Marta, too, acknowledged that the important point is to continue to surround the honesty with a positive perspective: "I tend to be very matter-of-fact because the first question [Frankie] will ask is, 'Owwie?' I say, 'Yeah, there'll be a bit of an owwie, and we'll get through it'" (personal communication, December 19, 2015).

Despite the anxiety associated with a painful procedure, parents do a disservice to their children if they are not honest. Nicole, Peter's mother, explained, "Oh, I explain to him exactly what's going on, like they're going to fix your palate because there's still a hole in it—he knows what his palate is—so, your speech is clearer" (personal communication, December 17, 2015).

Through honest communication painted in a positive manner with supporting contextual information, children are better able to navigate their medical situation and construct an understanding. However, care must be taken because too much information can backfire; instead of helping to create consonance, further anxiety and dissonance is possible (Jaaniste et al., 2007; Fernandes et al., 2014). Marta has learned this to be very true and explained that she now waits until right before a procedure when Frankie arrives at pre-admission or the pre-op area to begin preparing her for what is about to happen. "Prior to that, I don't because we have a lot of anxiety issues and those just take over. I find if I give too much preparation it really backfires on us" (Marta, personal communication, December 19, 2015).

Motivated to avoid this very scenario with Bethany, Paula and George have coined the family phrase: "We're going to fix this small problem so we don't get big problems" (George, personal communication, December 19, 2015). They have combined positivity with a lesser amount of information, which they feel is more appropriate for Bethany and what she is able to handle. In this, Bethany is given an opportunity to successfully construct understanding that breeds trust with her parents and caretakers.

Symbols of Comfort

In addition to information shared, items of comfort were shown to indirectly communicate reassurance. In moments when children cannot ask questions of or interact with those from whom they desire to gain information, they can experience security through an object that represents a significant relationship. For Victor, this item is his blanket and two favorite stuffed animals for surgeries. "He'll want his blanket on him. . . . So, I ask [the nurses] after they put their blanket on to put his blanket over. [So when] he wakes up, he feels the blanket" (Cindy, personal communication, January 5, 2016).

Linda shared that she often suggests that Brooks bring items from home to help him feel comfortable while at the hospital. She also offers to give him massages or something new to bring. "I always ask him to get like a new pajama or a new pillow—something special for him" (Linda, personal communication, January 10, 2016).

Some children's hospitals have pet therapy programs that bring trained dogs into children's rooms while they are inpatient. Carol told me that Jacob enjoys it when the dogs visit. During my time talking with Jacob, he began to shut down and not want to talk about his experiences with surgery or going to visit his doctors in their clinics. However, when I followed up with the question of whether he likes the doggies in the hospital, he immediately perked up with excitement and told me, "Yes!" (Jacob, personal communication, December 18, 2015). He told me the doggies help him not be scared.

Taylor developed quite an attachment to Stuffies, a specific type of stuffed animal. Following one of her very first surgeries, Taylor's grandmother brought her a Stuffy that made noise when it was squeezed. Because of the type of cranial facial surgery, Taylor could not open her eyes; however, the noise of the Stuffy brought such delight to Taylor. "They make me feel happy. They're soft and cuddly" (Taylor, personal communication, December 31, 2015). Since then she has gathered quite the collection of Stuffies.

Stuffed animals are also a source of comfort for Frankie and Reagan. For Frankie, it is her oversized bear, Ethan. Marta told me he often tags along to clinic appointments in addition to surgical procedures. Frankie brought him to the living room where we were chatting and nurtured him much like a mother would with her child. She also was sure to point out that Ethan was included in her drawing of her in the operating room (see Appendix B, Frankie).

Reagan, too, drew and explained that she took stuffed animals with her for a source of comfort (see Reagan's drawing in Appendix B). She often requires the medical staff to demonstrate what the procedure is like on the stuffed animals prior to performing it on her. This demonstration of the use of a familiar item from home not only reveals how it brings a sense of security and comfort, but how it also can be a tool by which the medical staff could build a relationship and establish communication channels that lessen anxiety on the part of the child and bring about more assurance.

Regardless of whether the children actively or passively seek information about physical implications, the process, or the end result, there is significance in the way by which understanding is constructed. Relationships with people and items can directly impact this process and determine to which information sources children turn.

Chapter 4

Looking for Information in Not So Likely Sources

A Case for Medically Themed Media

Parents, medical staff, and other caretakers are sources who can provide information in a direct fashion. This is often through question and answer periods. However, the communication with medical staff and caretakers is often complicated by procedures and time constraints. Each child in this book acknowledged the consistent presence of his or her parent(s) and the need for it.

Reagan's words "Because you guys are right there with me" (personal communication, January 20, 2016) hit me. Prior to my sitting down with her and formally asking her about her thoughts regarding her medical experience, she had never verbally expressed the impact that her daddy's and my presence had on her. When so much seems to be spinning out of these children's control, the stability of parental presence is meaningful (Filova & Sikorova, 2015; Whiting, 2009). Much like how Peter deeply desired his mom's presence—and used the routine request for her to bring him a Popsicle to ensure she stayed close by, Reagan relied on my husband and I to be there for her and to provide information when she did not even know how to form a question.

This was also true for Victor. His drawing of himself at the hospital included himself, a doctor, and his mommy. When I asked him where his mommy was, he replied, "Mommy is *very* close," (Victor, personal communication, January 5, 2016). He then told me her being by his side made him happy.

Earlier it was noted that trust was a significant factor in children's passive construction of understanding. Taylor's dependence on her parents for asking questions and being her source of information showed her trust. In talking with her she explained to me that without her parents she could only "sort of understand" what the doctors told her (Taylor, personal communication, December 31, 2015).

While every child acknowledged the important role these people play, especially parents, Leslie was honest and told me while she loved her mommy and wanted her close by, it did not help take the pain away. She, of course, would have been far more insecure without her mom, "but it didn't work because I was still scared. I keep crying and it keeps on hurting" (Leslie, personal communication, January 10, 2016). In moments like these, indirect communication methods such as medical play, visuals, and narratives can be resourceful.

Indirect information sources provide children with tools by which they can observe, and in essence overhear, information about their medical situations (Craddock, 2002). In such, information and truth are realized when children inwardly relate that which they see and hear to their own experience (Kierkegaard, 1846/1992). Knowledge may not be formally assembled, but the insights gained indirectly inform a child's life (Coles, 1990). Children can relate with a character's struggle to be accepted by peers or the innate desire for love and acceptance. When characters in narratives or medical play experience a renewed sense of self-worth, children, too, can sense the feeling of belonging.

MEDICAL PLAY

The narrative paradigm mirrors human life. It is through this relationship that narrative becomes so compelling. MacIntyre (1981) posits, "The criteria for success or failure in a human life as a whole are the criteria of success or failure in a narrated or to-be-narrated quest" (p. 203). As stories are told, culture is impacted because people's thoughts, opinions, and beliefs are affected (Hunt, 2003). Children are capable of enjoying all the wonder narrated characters and plots can hold while recognizing how their life story relates to that which is being narrated; the children internalize the truths of a story. Kierkegaard (1846/1992) claims that the secrets within stories are only influential because of their subjectivity: "Inwardness is truth" (p. 300).

The use of dolls and toy medical equipment allows children to observe how various medical tools are used; the intimate details of their journey including degrees of invasion of personal space, touch, and pain can be realized and even negotiated. Because children innately seek ways to master stress through the gathering of information and construction of understanding, play therapy provides a way for feelings to be expressed and energy released in a spontaneous fashion (Le Roy et al., 2003). During such play, children's emotions can be monitored while also assessing their ability to understand the information indirectly presented about their medical situation. Children are afforded more control as they, too, perform the task at hand. In this medical play, children are made to feel less alone and as if someone else is also experiencing the procedure.

Peter was given a doll to keep before his last surgery. "He got to draw the face on it. He put the numbing cream on the doll. He gave the doll the IV; he gave the doll a needle! That was a huge help. . . . This surgery was supposed to be more painful than the other one, and he responded better" (Nicole, personal communication, December 17, 2015). Nicole believes playing out the procedure of anesthesia on the doll greatly minimized Peter's anxiety.

The idea of role-play also helped Hannah as she has grown and become more aware of the discomfort involved with trache changes. "We had the (respiratory therapist) from home care come and she had a doll with a trache in it that she used for teaching purposes. [Hannah] got so attached to this doll that she had to have one of her own. So, I had to buy her a doll, and I had to put the old trache into it" (Cara, personal communication, December 20, 2015). Hannah's attachment to the doll indirectly signals a relationship of acceptance; there is a doll that looks like her.

Marta explained that medical play has provided Frankie the space and time she needs to make sense of her experiences. "She often wants Stollery [Hospital] baby shirts to put on her babies, and then it's fascinating to watch the medical play that she does. . . . If someone comes over, it's all medical play. And you can just see that that's her processing" (Marta, personal communication, December 19, 2015). Although Marta recalled a time Frankie heard a storybook read and took the idea of medical play a little too literally: "It's called *Jesse's Journey*, I think. It's about this kid also getting a g-tube. She literally took her doll, cut her belly open and tried to put a g-tube right in. I'm like, 'Wow! We're really taking this to a new level'" (personal communication, December 19, 2015). Both Marta and I shared a laugh and concurred that the silver lining was that it was only a doll.

VISUAL AND NARRATIVE RHETORIC

Frankie's story above, though, is a great example of the rhetorical power that pictures and stories can have. Narrative's indirect communication permits children to become engaged in a world not their own. By being privy to another's life, conversation, and actions, children overhear powerful hegemonic lessons. Many families in this study either have used photos, social stories (e.g., a description using narrative and visual techniques in order to share social information about a situation or skill), or various children's storybooks and television shows to present children with information about their experiences. "Simple explanations are okay, but I think pictures with a social story are much better—because it's a visual and a story" (Nicole, personal communication, December 17, 2015).

When Kyler received his stuffed moose, Vibe, at the Cochlear convention it came with a coloring book. At the time he knew very little about what a BAHA hearing aide would look like and do for him. "[The book] kind of introduces [Vibe] and kind of explains to [Kyler] in a kid-way what's going on in terms of the hearing loss" (Chris, personal communication, January 10, 2016). As Kyler got older, he appreciated the story and the stuffed moose more. When I asked him what is so cool about Vibe's story, Kyler told me: "That he has (hearing aides) without a band" (personal communication, January 10, 2016). At the time of the interview, Kyler had one bandless BAHA, which was placed during his first aesthetic ear reconstructive surgery, with the second one scheduled in about six months.

Nathan, Jacob, and Frankie use augmented communication devices. Within these machines there are programs and/or apps that combine photos with social stories to help children better visualize and construct an understanding about an upcoming situation or procedure. "If you do this, this is what happens; if you do that, that's what happens" (Nicole, personal communication, December 17, 2015). The visual reference is a source offering information regarding predictability.

During one of Reagan's lengthy hospital stays, her auntie gave her a very large stuffed lion. Reagan named the lion "Brave Dave." Since that hospital stay, Brave Dave has accompanied Reagan on many procedures and surgeries. As a family, we have made up hospital adventures for Brave Dave and Reagan; we have pretended that they are super heroes and can be brave through the many procedures they face. I put these adventures into narrative form with the help of a friend who drew some illustrations. We keep a digital version on Reagan's iPad, and she reads her Brave Dave story before almost every procedure. She told me her favorite adventure was when "you pretend to go in a car" instead of simply rolling down a hallway in her hospital bed (Reagan, personal communication, January 20, 2016). The affinity Reagan has with Brave Dave and the story provides a familiar reference by which medical situations can be contextualized. This concept extends into Bandura's (1971) social cognitive theory.

Albert Bandura (1971) first developed social learning theory that focused on how ideologies are constructed and behaviors are learned based on observation modeling within a social system. The theory would become social cognitive theory as Bandura (1982) added the emphasis on social reinforcement of behavior. Bandura's (1971, 1982, 2001) idea of self-efficacy correlates with an individual's confidence in the ability to model specific behaviors. In light of these children's medical experiences, these behaviors can include acts of bravery modeled by socially meaningful characters (Lauricella et al.,

2011). With this theory in mind, the interviews with the children suggest that the usefulness of visual and narrative information sources come from the children's abilities to observe another child or character in a similar situation, assess the behavior and its results, and compare how it relates to their situation.

MEDICALLY THEMED MEDIA

For children who live in a constant state of anticipation of what and when the next painful procedure might be, there exists a great need for resources to help them make sense of their experiences. The expectancy of pain and sensitivity to anxiety can have considerable and concurrent effects (Kennedy et al., 2011). Much of these children's struggles come from navigating the pain and anxiety coupled with uncertainty. These children can regain consonance when they are afforded specific information.

Just as Lauricella et al. (2011) have purported, media or media content that are socially meaningful can have great affect. The very nature of it makes it highly rhetorical for the sense-making processes of children who are engaged in experiences associated with their difficult medical journeys. "It's all about communication and about how much is communicated and how it's communicated" (Cara, personal communication, December 20, 2015).

Therefore, medically themed media not only can provide information using visual and narrative strategies making them highly rhetorical, but also offer parents and medical caretakers more appropriate means by which to help these children understand and make sense of their experiences. While this is highly desirable for all those involved in pediatric care, it is a fairly new concept. Having an effective tool intentionally created to meet children's information and sense-making needs is critical. "It's about how comfortable you've made the parents feel [so] that they can in turn bring that forward to their kids" (Cara, personal communication, December 20, 2015).

For example, when Leslie broke her arm she made the connection between her x-rays and one of her favorite films, *Pirates of the Caribbean.* Like the movie, Leslie called her x-rays, "Ooooh, stinky bones" (personal communication, January 10, 2016). Kim told me that Leslie thought the x-rays were the coolest things; the *Pirates of the Caribbean* tie helped eliminate anxiety and moved the appointments along. They used the same principle for other procedures; whether it was a story or show, they tried to relate it to other medical procedures so she could better understand.

Carol had seen the impact of visuals and narratives on Jacob. "He just seems to be a little bit calmer" (Carol, personal communication, December 18, 2015). Jacob had particularly grown attached to Nickelodeon's *Bubble*

Guppies children's television series. He especially liked the first episode titled *The Clambulance*, which is a perfect example of medically themed media as previously discussed. Carol described the show: "Avi's hurt, but it's okay because they're going to get him taken care of. There's no fake 'everything will be okay,' but everyone's calm about it. They all have their jobs to do and they [do them]" (personal communication, December 18, 2015).

USEFULNESS AND IMPACT

The examples of children being drawn to medically themed media, especially Jacob, Leslie, and Reagan's, suggest usefulness. Bethany, too, explained how she thought it would be fun for some of her favorite books or shows to incorporate sleep studies. She shared how the two main characters, which are twins, in her favorite *Disney Channel* show, *Liv and Maddie,* often switch places to benefit themselves depending on the situation. "Well, I think her twin sister, Liv, would do a switcheroony where Liv does the sleep study and Maddie just lives her day" (Bethany, personal communication, December 19, 2015).

As mentioned earlier, Bethany has an affinity with the book, *Put Me In The Zoo.* She explained to me that she would change the storyline to include the animals saying, "You can't put me in the sleep study" (Bethany, personal communication, December 19, 2015). In spite of Bethany's noted tendencies to not want to discuss her medical situation, the questions asking for her thoughts of what experiences medically themed media could include encouraged a lot of discussion from Bethany. It was through this framing of our conversation that the potential of medically themed media to have influential and sense-making value was shown.

While every parent said they supported the idea of medically themed media, Cindy, Victor's mother, suggested that the media use children instead of animals or other imaginary creatures within the narratives. She gave the example of the *Disney Junior Channel's Kate and Mim-Mim* show and drew attention to the connections Victor made with Kate when she appears to interact with other human beings rather than when Kate interacts with Mim-Mim and other imaginary characters: "He responds to real children, maybe animated children, but it'd have to be like no talking stuffed animals; it'd have to be like real families" (Cindy, personal communication, January 5, 2016).

Marta also noted her observed benefits of using real people. Frankie's connection with the Miracle Child videos was in the narrative being told, but also in her ability to easily relate to the featured children and their stories.

"It was real life. It was real events, and they did a great job" (Marta, personal communication, December 19, 2015). Perhaps young children connect more strongly with prosocial messages when they are indirectly communicated using depictions of real people.

Linda, Brooks' mother, also supported the narrative nature of medically themed media that allows room for indirect communication. She explained that she wished the surgeon's online videos that Brooks watched prior to his first surgery were more cartoon in nature: "It's too hard for them to see the real situation" (personal communication, January 10, 2016).

Earlier Brooks' drawing of himself and the doctor just prior to surgery (see Appendix B, Brooks) was discussed in light of the possibility that children feel lonely as they navigate their medical journey. After Linda, Brooks' mother, saw his drawing and heard his description of being alone, she shared her surprise because the picture Brooks drew did not represent her being with him. "He's picturing his situation more how the videos were" (Linda, personal communication, January 10, 2016). Linda shared that while the videos helped Brooks understand the process of his surgery, giving him reassurance that he, too, would have a complete real-looking ear, she believed her son would have benefited more from an animated narrative.

Indeed narratives have the power to help children make sense of their medical journeys. Cara, Hannah's mother, also stated that she felt if parents were more comfortable with information surrounding their children's care, they would be better equipped to explain it and engage with their child. Perhaps medically themed media could be a tool to bridge conversation between the parent and child. "I think [medically themed media] would be helpful as long as we incorporate them into our discussions" (Cara, personal communication, December 20, 2015).

The use of medically themed media might also provide time and space for children to process the difficulty of their situation, understand the procedures and potential results, in addition to their ability to be resilient throughout the navigation of their medical journey. Carol shared that after every doctor's appointment, procedure, or trip to the hospital Jacob wanted to watch his favorite *Bubble Guppies* episode, *The Clambulance*:

> You can see that the wheels are turning and that he is thinking about it. And even though his expressive communication is so low compared to his receptive, he gets it and it gets him processing it. Especially when the media or the story has—you don't want to say positive because this is not always going to be positive, but if it's as well-handled as possible, as calm as possible, as "this is how it's going to be and everyone's doing this to make sure that you feel better" sort of thing in as caring a way as possible, I think the potential is huge for it. (personal communication, December 18, 2015)

THE NEED FOR MORE AWARENESS

No matter the genre of media, the examples above point to the impact that media as an information source, especially those with medical themes, can have on children's construction of understanding. The visual nature of most medically themed media increases their rhetorical influence because children favor information presented in a visual manner. While every parent praised the idea of medically themed media, most quickly stated that they were unfamiliar with anything that would be appropriate for their child's medical journey. The following comments show the support for but lack of awareness regarding the idea of medically themed media:

- "Absolutely, I think it would be great for a kid to see just so things aren't so unfamiliar. So, if they do hear the beeping noise, they're like, 'Oh yeah; that's the same one that I heard before.' For sure, I think that would be fabulous" (Amy, Taylor's mother, personal communication, December 31, 2015).
- "[Medically themed media] have never even crossed my mind, [but] words mean nothing to this child. He needs the visual" (Cindy, Victor's mother, personal communication, January 5, 2016).
- "I think if I knew that there were those resources available I would. I haven't come across any and I haven't been told of any" (Cara, Hannah's mother, personal communication, December 20, 2015).
- "No I haven't [come across any medically themed media], but she probably would benefit because her class, they use lots of visuals" (Nicole, Nadia's mother, personal communication, December 17, 2015).
- "No, I guess I could say be strong like BayMax or something, but in the moment I'm just trying to get him through" (Roxanne, Wyatt's mother, personal communication, December 10, 2015).

The children expressed a great liking of various books, television shows, movies, or characters, but only five participating families referenced media with specific medical content. As noted above, Jacob's favorite show to watch is *The Clambulance* episode of *Bubble Guppies.* His mom, Carol, shared that he must identify with it:

> Yeah, I think he might just because he keeps going to it after every single time we go to the doctor, every time we have a trache change or anything like that. He's always referring to that one, so there must be something in that whole program that he finds soothing. (personal communication, December 18, 2015)

When Reagan was asked what comfort items she took with her to the hospital she immediately stated, "The hospital friends book" (personal communication, January 20, 2016). She was referencing the *Berenstain Bears* book titled, *Hospital Friends*, which is a story about Brother and Sister Bear taking a tour of the hospital and making friends with other bears who work there. This book was a fairly new acquisition to her collection of children's books, but it was the book she asked to bring with her during her last emergency room visit for possible shunt failure. In response to the question of why she especially liked bringing that book, Reagan added, "Mama, Papa, Sister, and Brother are in it and because you guys are right there with me" (personal communication, January 20, 2016). Reagan recognized the relationships, the togetherness, and the stability of the Bear family in the book; those concepts held significant meaning for her and brought comfort in spite of so much uncertainty and the inability to predict the process of procedures.

Frankie routinely watches online videos titled, *Miracle Child*, that have documented the incredible journeys of various children who have been treated at the Stollery Children's Hospital. She was featured in one of the videos and watched that episode quite a bit. "You can just see her getting joy out of that" (Marta, personal communication, December 19, 2015).

Brooks and Kyler also talked about the videos their plastic surgeon had produced and made available online for their viewing prior to surgery. The videos were direct in nature with explanations and real images of the procedure; there was no narrative that would enable the child to "overhear" the process and goals of their aesthetic ear reconstruction surgeries. Kyler's parents felt the videos were helpful for their son. Linda, too, was supportive of the idea.

Regardless of the families' awareness, use of high-profile medically themed media, or primitive creation of personal sources, they all agreed the idea of having and using them was exceptional. Paula, Bethany's mother, noted that the indirect communication style afforded by medical play and medically themed media was an appealing idea because the information is presented "without bringing it constantly to somebody's attention" (personal communication, December 19, 2015). She added, "If you have a scab and you're always picking at it, it's always at your attention and the scab is not getting better. So it's a matter of that balance of [providing information that answers their questions and allows for] healing and seeing positive results without it always being out there" (Paula, personal communication, December 19, 2015). These families expressed desire for more high-profile and popular medically themed media to be created.

LOOKING AHEAD

The limited use of and yet high interest in medically themed media preliminarily support the notion of their rhetorical influence on helping children to make sense of their medical experiences while also modeling behaviors that can help to restore consonance. Medically themed media can be a powerful tool to meet hospitalized children's information needs. In light of this, there is a great call to those who fund children's healthcare supportive technologies to invest in the creation of medically themed media that specifically targets young children with imaginative visual representations of their very real medical struggles.

Medically themed media can in fact be the means of providing suggestions that, as Bettelheim (1975/2010) put it, come in symbolic form and best help children work through difficulty into maturity. Together with such funding sources, media creators would do well to develop medically themed media that is just as successful and socially meaningful as other major children's programming, such as *Disney* or *Nickelodeon.* In so doing, it would be interesting to consider the impact of using characters represented as children instead of make-believe figures (e.g., talking animals, monsters, extraterrestrial characters, etc.) while including multiple stories that depict a variety of medical experiences.

Parents need greater access to information resources to help their children construct understanding and make sense of their difficult situations. While families often consult their physicians for information, they also turn to the Internet but are often left to create their own devices in order to communicate meaning in a way that is appropriate for their children. The more parents use visual and narrative elements, the more effective the communication of information can be. Just as Bettelheim (1975/2010) likened the fairy tale to a medium that offers life solutions through imagination in a way that children can understand, medically themed media can also enlighten children regarding certain beliefs, values, and behaviors that offer greater meaning throughout their medical journeys. Through medically themed media's ability to model such behaviors, restoration of consonance, sense-making, and the development of resiliency are witnessed.

Chapter 5

Conclusion

This research was inspired by the realization that the information needs of children have been largely understudied, especially outside of pediatric oncology contexts. Additionally, it was originally birthed out of observing my own daughter's sense-making journey and my family's desire to meet her information needs. That personal exploration led to the desire to investigate the experiences of other children and the processes by which they constructed an understanding of their medical situations.

Throughout this book there is considerable inquiry of what these children's information needs are and how they might be met. It also specifically considered children's use of medically themed media as an information source. For children with difficult medical experiences, their attempt to make sense of their situations is at the core of their communication behavior. Whether it was Bethany's vivid remembrance of the interior design of her sleep study's room, Hannah's memory of exactly what her anesthesiologist was wearing, or Frankie's recall of a seizure she had had four years prior when revisiting the store in her local mall in which the seizure had taken place, these children are distinctly aware of their surroundings and desire to construct an understanding in order to make sense of their experiences.

These children recognize that pain and difficulty are involved and in spite of the routine nature of their medical care, they still desire to find ways to resist the difficulty and lessen the pain. Hannah's drawing, as shown in Appendix B, reveals how familiarity is acknowledged, but does not make the situation desirable; when asked about what could make the situation easier, Hannah said, "Nothing" (personal communication, December 20, 2015). Preparation for any hospital visit or procedure is crucial; both Nicole, Nathan's mother, and Marta, Frankie's mother, shared how giving their children time to process what each step of the treatment plan would entail was critical for their children's sense-making abilities. The children also desired to know what the end result would be. With the knowledge that he would be able to have clearer speech, Peter did much better managing his anxiety as he prepared for his cleft lip and palate surgery. Ultimately, these children desire to know how their procedures will affect them.

The research contained within this book increases the importance of all contentions calling for sensitivity in a healthcare approach that considers a broad viewpoint of the grand role that even one procedure plays in the larger scope of children's treatment plans. For example, Carol, Jacob's mother, declared, "[I wish other healthcare professionals would better understand] how much it impacts their daily lives. Because for care like our kids, it's not just a one-time 'I'm scared to go to the dentist' sort-of-thing. It bleeds into every minute of every day" (personal communication, December 18, 2015). For children exemplified by those in this book, the medical procedures can be many. The constant role of sense-making must be recognized in children's construction of understanding and the information sources they access.

Therefore, it is incumbent upon parents and caretakers to find and utilize information resources that do not distract from and attempt to dismiss the pain and confusion of a situation but rather help these children to navigate their medical journey. Cara poignantly stated, "Touching somebody by connecting with their emotions and their feelings is a big thing" (personal communication, December 20, 2015). Children also need information resources that help them construct an understanding of their medical situations in a manner that sensitively considers their greater journey about who they are in spite of the difficulty involved. Flannery O'Connor (1979) penned the rather appropriate line: "In a sense sickness is a place, more instructive than a long trip to Europe, and it's always a place where nobody can follow" (p. 163). The sense these children make of their medical experiences is unique and profound.

The burden for the creation and study of medically themed media may never have been greater. This in fact points to a new type of relationship between communication and psychology research as medically themed media provide an indirect way of communicating security to these children. Indeed psychology research is well-established within healthcare contexts with a large focus on the understanding of fear and its sources (Freud, 1920), the use of preparation and coping techniques to assist with the management of fear and pain (Melamed et al., 1976; Melamed et al., 1983; Mahajan et al., 1998; King et al., 2001; Cohen et al., 2002; Langer et al., 2005; Field, 2006), identity construction and peer interaction when diagnoses are disclosed (Meyerson, 1948; Tajfel, 1978; Tajfel & Turner, 1985; La Greca & Bearman, 2000; Stets & Burke, 2000; Alderfer et al., 2001), and information needs of patients specifically dealing with cancer (Ellis & Leventhal, 1993; Hooker,

1997; Mitchell et al., 2006; Mitchell, 2012). Meanwhile Bandura (2001) is perhaps most noted for establishing the connection between media and behavioral modeling; McLuhan (1964) and Kuhn (1985) also established the social and psychological affect of media on human behavior while Lauricella et al. (2011) and Strouse & Troseth (2008) discovered that when video is found to be socially meaningful there is psychological and behavioral impact. However, only a handful of scholars have considered the use of media as an effective psychological tool for navigating through and coping with medical diagnoses and treatments (Pinto & Hollandsworth, 1989; Schmitt et al., 1999; Fernandes et al., 2014). Yet none of these studies have considered the use of high-profile and popular medically themed media.

Opportunities for meaningful scholarly research in this area of study are many and greatly needed. Many questions remain regarding how greater awareness of medically themed media of various types might influence the effectiveness of children's sense-making and their ability to construct understanding of their medically related experiences.

The findings presented within this book also bring insight to the information needs of children who face routine medical procedures. Perhaps the notion that children desire to know the physical implications of a procedure, the process it will entail, and what the end result will be can lay a foundation upon which media creators base content production. Research regarding the influence of such media on hospitalized children is needful.

Another aspect of medically themed media that would be interesting to consider further is the use of children as characters versus animals or other imaginary characters. Cindy, Victor's mother, shared that media with animals or imaginary characters hold no significant meaning to him; however, media messages that use children do in fact resonate. This notion warrants further exploration.

This book did not specifically explore the relationship between children's information needs and coping abilities. While some coping characteristics such as hope, security, and resiliency were mentioned, this area of research would benefit from future studies that more closely explore coping. It would be especially interesting to consider coping in light of medically themed media's impact.

This research pioneers a new consideration of both the importance of meaningful information sources for children and children's media within the healthcare context that includes a large variety of diagnoses and experiences beyond those of oncology patients. The rhetorical narratives within medically themed media can establish a foundation for these children's understanding of what a procedure's physical implications, process, and final outcome will be. With this knowledge and the modeling of sense-making and resilient behaviors, these children can begin restoring consonance as they are afforded the opportunity to process through their difficult situations and construct an understanding of what their journey entails and the resiliency that is within them. After all, the one procedure they find themselves presently experiencing is likely not their first and it will not be their last.

Appendix A

A Note on My Research Methods

Because of Reagan's journey, I am most familiar with this grouping of diagnoses and the procedures these patients experience. Additionally, my involvement in the craniofacial community allowed for easier access to hearing other patients and families' stories. Each family gave permission for the disclosure of its members' names and the details of their lived experiences. It is their hope that other families may benefit through a general greater awareness of children's sense-making and information needs.

I desired to make a compassionate space for the overwhelming threads of what may feel as an untamable fabric within these children's lives. I wanted to hear each child's story and understand their raw emotions that come with the fearful procedures; I wanted to grasp this information while ensuring that the struggle of these children and their families was not misrepresented. To do this, I relied heavily on input from the children's parents, interviews with the children, which incorporated drawings, and field observations.

ETHNOGRAPHIC APPROACH

Face-to-face interviews with each child and their parents provided invaluable insight. The input attained from the parents provided a breadth of knowledge pertaining to the background of each child's diagnosis and treatment journey, in addition to the effectiveness of information sources. Yet, a richer understanding was possible through the pairing of parent responses with the children's descriptions of their lived experiences (Mishler, 1986). It was also important to use in-depth semi-structured interviews to help the children build their own narratives regarding how they make sense of their experiences and the role that various information sources, including medically themed media, play in this. "The goal in narrative interviewing is to generate detailed accounts rather than brief answers or general statements" (Riessman, 2008, p. 23). Elements of Brenda Dervin's Sense-Making Methodology and Micro-Moment Time-Line Interviewing (MMTLI) provided for these in-depth accounts.

Sense-making is about communication behavior. As a methodology, it recognizes that reality is never complete, nor constant, but is conceptualized as situational (Dervin, 2003a). However, gaps or discontinuities in understanding inhibit the immediacy of the sense-making process. In order for individuals to make sense of their situation, they must gather information and construct understanding in order to fill the existing gap (Dervin, 1983). Dervin (1983) refers to this as the situation-gap-use model. Dervin, Foreman-Wernet, and Lauterbach (2003) expanded the model to place greater emphasis on the gap and a bridging that helps to compensate for it. I drew on this bridging idea and asked the parents and children to describe their situations, the gaps they face, the ways in which they construct bridges, and how they picture their outcome. In order to bring about various ideas, thoughts, feelings, and emotions that led to sense-making, Dervin (2008) stressed the importance of empowering interviewees to guide the storytelling process. This was done through means related to MMTLI.

The MMTLI process was designed to focus on specific moments in time-space that participants believe to be significant. As these moments were described, particular care was taken to probe into the gaps they face, the bridges they construct, and the outcomes they experience. Interviewees intentionally led the discussion so that the conversation flowed from their "mind's eye" while the interviewer remained as objective as possible in thought or reaction to what is described (Dervin, 1992; 2003c).

It is fitting that Dervin (2003b) acknowledged the successful use of MMTLI with "cancer patients, blood donors, internal medicine patients, college students, disabled adults, children, low-income and general population adults, and Asian refugees" (p. 257). The prior success with people living on the margins of life supported my application of this method with children in medical situations. MMTLI "ask[ed] informants to describe their sense-makings and sense-unmakings as they occurred in the 'time-line steps' of a given situation" (Dervin, 2008, p. 23). This study defined the "given situation" as a child's particular medical experience that demonstrates possible fear and sense-making techniques.

Recognizing that children use multimodal ways to communicate, it was vital to be sensitive to how they might best tell about their lives (Anning & Ring, 2004; Kinnunen & Einarsdottir, 2013). The multimodal approach assumed that "meanings are made, distributed, received, interpreted, and remade in interpretation through many representational and communicative modes not just through language" (Kress & Jewitt, 2003, p. 1). Leitch (2008) posited that drawing allows children to narrate aspects of their lived experiences and uncover "unsayable" stories. The MMTLI process was adapted to include drawing as a means to assist the children in actively communicating and constructing their reality.

McKay and Kendrick (2001) noted that the use of questions help to stimulate children's drawings. Liamputtong and Fernandes (2015) also purported a research method of using prompts with children as they draw but also asking them to describe what they have drawn; the describing process allows for further probing and connections to be made about situations, gaps, and uses for sense-making. "Moreover, for participants to describe their drawing necessitates reflection not only on the drawing but also on the relationship of what they have drawn to their particular [situation] and the significance of what they have drawn to their previous statements" (Guillemin, 2004, p. 277).

Combined with MMTLI, children were asked to draw their experiences (see Appendix B). The drawings underlined the value of the stories told by the children participating in this study. They provided insight into the multimodal ways in which children narrate their experiences and construct meaning. I used this combination, in addition to observation, to help break down barriers and make the children more comfortable while allowing powerful space for their insights and emotions about medical experiences and coping techniques to be expressed. Each child was provided with a box of crayons and a drawing pad to keep following the interview.

PARENT AS RESEARCHER

Goodall (2000) described reflexivity as "careful thought that is informed by existing scholarly thinking in addition to whatever personal passages are folded into the reflective passages" (p. 38). The numerous scholarly sources cited throughout this project support Goodall's point. However, this study was birthed out of a personal experience and passion to hopefully help other hospitalized children and their parents make sense of their medical journeys. Similarly, Seidman (2006) found that "at the heart of interviewing research is an interest in other individuals' stories because they are of worth" (p. 9).

I contend that my personal experience added to the validity of this study, especially in that I brought a deep level of genuine interest in and intimate knowledge related to the topic (Beyer, 1992; Denzin & Lincoln, 1994). Additionally, Adler and Adler (1997) noted that the role of parent-as-researcher provides access to the group being studied while the researcher would otherwise appear out of place. For me, I never stop being a "medical mama." I regularly frequent clinical and hospital settings and talk about my daughter's test and image results with doctors. I know all too well the discussions of preparing a child for the next treatment or procedure. Because of my role as a "medical mama," it was natural for me to become immersed in the world of each participant.

RESEARCH SAMPLE

This study focused on children aged three to thirteen years because they have specific vulnerabilities to fear and distress that are compounded by their age, access—or the lack thereof—to resources, and lack of control (Blount, Powers, Cotter, Swan, and Free, 1994); they also are beginning to make sense of their world (Buckingham, 1993, 2003; Potter, 2005; Schmitt, Anderson, & Collins, 1999). "This ontogenesis is assisted by others providing concepts through language, and stimulation to growth through interaction" (Bruner & Haste, 2011, p. 6).

The children include seven males and seven females for a total of 14 participants. For each of these children, at least one parent agreed to also participate. In order for these children to qualify as participants, they had to be patients undergoing treatment for craniofacial, neurological, or neurosurgical anomalies and be between three and thirteen years of age. This age range was important in selecting children whose coping techniques have largely been understudied (Fernandes, Arriaga, & Esteves, 2014). Additionally, the selected age range was appropriate as parents, caretakers, and healthcare professionals often have difficulty with explaining unfamiliar procedures, diagnoses, and equipment in ways that help younger children understand (Langer et al., 2005). Careful attention was given to participants' emotional states, cognitive abilities, and verbal skills to ensure the quality of the study and the well-being of the children participating remained intact.

With the help of personal contacts and an online support group, I identified children who fit the demographic criteria. My completion of HIPPA and medical research training assisted the opening of doors to make contact with the families. The interviews spanned two months between December 2015 and January 2016. The first group of interviews conducted for this study took place in Alberta, Canada, in December with one week until Christmas. While this study spans beyond the United States' borders to include Canada, a country with a healthcare system entirely run and supported by its government, the culture and experiences of the Canadian families did not vary from those of the families within the United States.

To gain access, I first contacted two parents who had participated in a previous study of mine and after securing their willingness to participate, I asked if they might have additional contacts. They put me in touch with one family via a Facebook support group. Upon my arrival and while interviewing families, newly suggested contacts were made. The six other children were recruited from Southern California by way of my relationships with special education teachers, medical professionals, or extracurricular activities. The two locations from which participants were recruited represent what became available to me.

While introducing myself to each family, I shared that I, too, was a parent of a child with a difficult medical journey. The families were inviting and willing to participate. Parents routinely told me that they hoped research like this study could make another family's navigation of difficult medical experiences easier. Family consent to participate was obtained before observation or interviews began. I observed the children to note any information-seeking behaviors. Their inquisition regarding my presence was also noted for any display of anxiety. Interviews, along with the children's drawings, were then conducted. Outside of my family, names have been changed to protect the participants' identities.

ANALYSIS

With the heart of this study being to explore the information needs of children who regularly encounter difficult medical procedures and examine their various information sources in their effort to make sense of their situation, 39 total hours were spent with the families producing nearly 15 hours of interview audio. Once these were transcribed and combined with field notes and the children's drawings (shown in Appendix B), more than 300 pages of data were available for analysis. This analysis revealed rich insight regarding the impact that these children's medical experiences were having on their ability to understand and make sense of life that is filled with uncertainty, difficulty, and yet somehow resiliency. Using the constant comparative method for coding and analyzing the data, which involved looking at the data in small "units" and working toward larger data sets (Lincoln & Guba, 1985; Silverman, 2011), a total of 44 recurring codes were recorded 752 times throughout the data. The codes were then sorted by topic and combined to reveal overarching themes discussed throughout this book.

Out of this, my goal was to provide readers with a rich description of the children's experiences. Beyond this description, I hoped to provide insight for the medical community to better come alongside and support the sense-making efforts of children, such as the ones that appear in this book, in order to help them face difficult medical procedures with less fear and greater understanding.

Appendix B

Children's Drawings

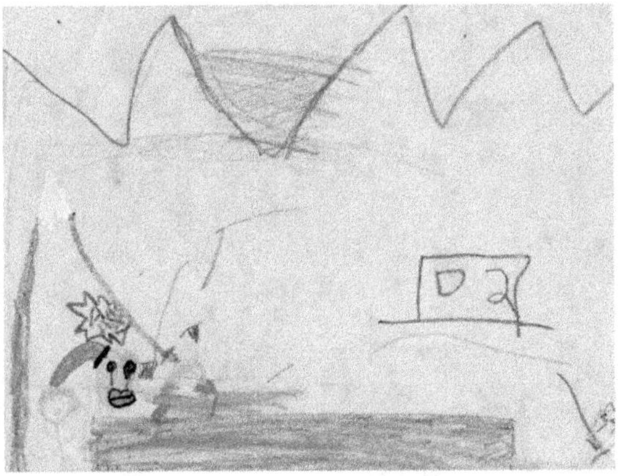

Figure B.1 Drawing by Bethany, 11. Her drawing of a sleep study depicts with so much detail her anxiety (e.g., thought bubble of screaming in her head and her tears) and her attempt to create consonance by drawing the technician relatively small in comparison to herself (personal communication, December 19, 2015).

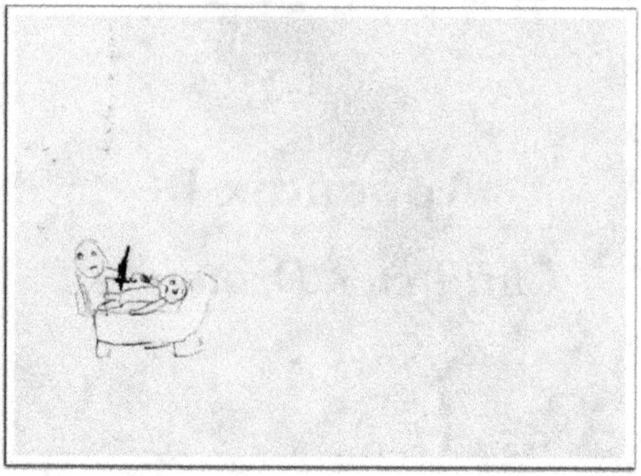

Figure B.2 Drawing by Brooks, 12. His drawing shows the difficulty he experienced during IV preparation prior to his surgery. Brooks explained that only he and the doctor were present, but Maria, Brooks' mother, stated that she was there, as well; she also suggested that Brooks likely remembered it only be him and the doctor due to the surgeon's preparatory information (personal communication, January 10, 2016). This showed Brooks' overwhelming sense of loneliness.

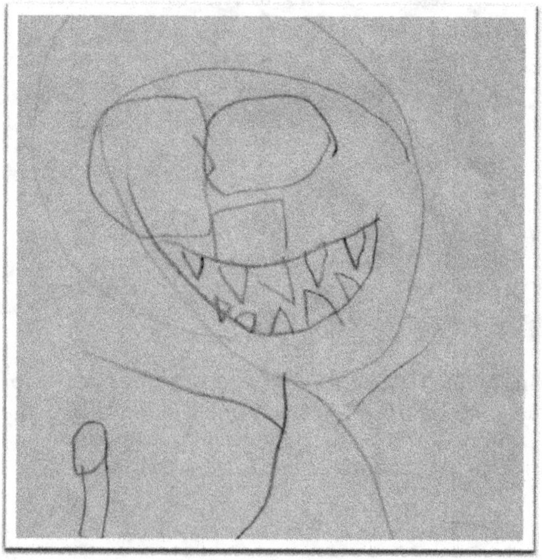

Figure B.3 Drawing by Frankie, 13. She drew herself undergoing her most recent dental surgery and refused to draw anything related to her anesthesia experience (e.g., the mask, IV, etc.), which was especially traumatic. Frankie did draw her bear, Ethan (drawn in the lower left corner), symbolizing the reassurance he brought her while she did not have the comfort of her mom's presence inside the operating room. Additionally, Frankie resisted drawing any of the medical staff; this suggested the consonance she desired to restore. However, she did state that the doctor helped her further showing her resilience (personal communication, December 19, 2015).

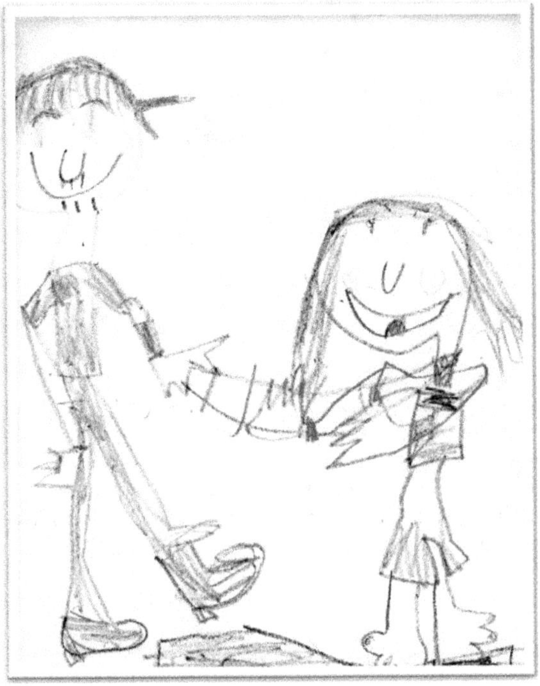

Figure B.4 Drawing by Hannah, 6. Her drawing included vivid detail of the anesthesiologist preparing her trache for surgery, including the articles of clothing and their details. While drawing she expressed that she does not like surgery, but that the familiarity with the process and her trust in the doctors helps her be resilient (personal communication, December 20, 2015).

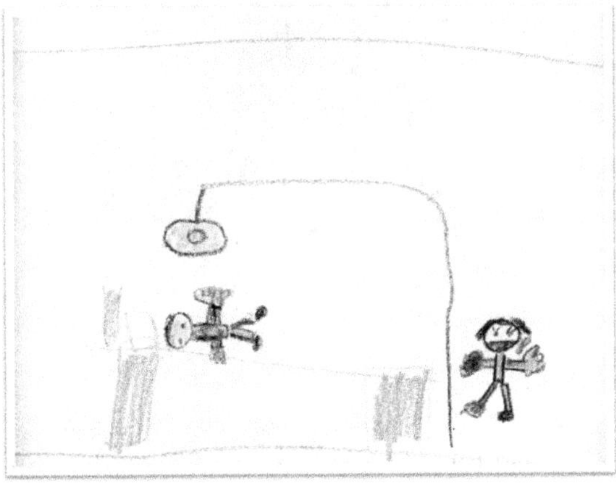

Figure B.5 Drawing by Kyler, 8. He drew himself in the middle of his ear reconstructive surgery. Only after completing this drawing and then being asked how he felt about this situation did he open up about the difficulty and fear he experienced (personal communication, January 10, 2016).

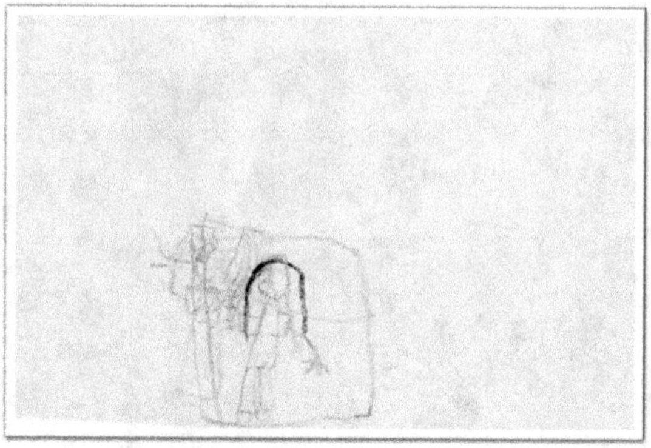

Figure B.6 Drawing by Leslie, 7. She drew her most recent difficult medical experience—the resetting of her broken arm. Leslie's body is clearly shown lying on the hospital table while a variety of machinery and medical staff attempt to align the bones within her arm. The resetting attempt was not successful. Leslie became emotional while talking about this experience; its difficulty made a significant impression on her (personal communication, January 10, 2016).

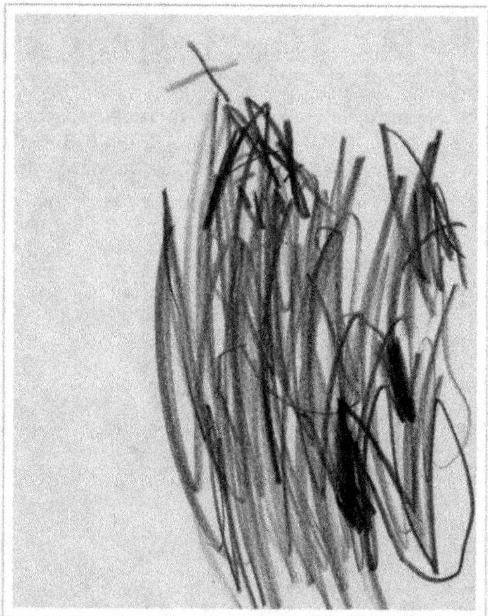

Figure B.7 Drawing by Peter, 5. His drawing began as nurses giving him an IV in the hospital prior to one of his cleft lip and palate surgeries. It is interesting that out of all color choices available in a 24-count crayon box, Peter chose black. As he was explaining the details of his picture, Peter adamantly colored over it and said that he was crying (personal communication, December 16, 2015). This clearly showed the difficulty of his experience and the consonance he desired to restore.

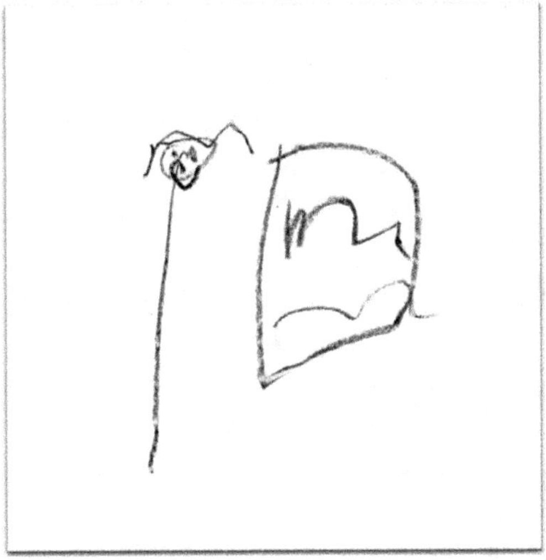

Figure B.8 Drawing by Reagan, 6. While she stated that she would draw herself during an MRI, she resisted drawing anything associated with the actual experience (e.g., preparation for the procedure, anesthesia, the long process, etc.) (personal communication, January 20, 2016). Instead, she focused on her leaving the MRI with happy anticipation for whatever rewards followed. This showed her desire for consonance. She also mentioned Disney Junior's Doc McStuffins' toys and how the added company is supportive during the difficult procedure.

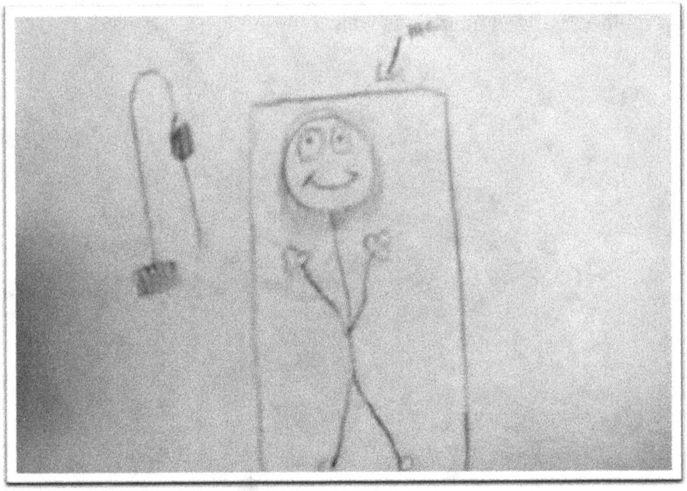

Figure B.9 Drawing by Taylor, 13. She drew herself lying on a hospital bed waking up from anesthesia after a surgery and before her parents were brought back to join her. Taylor explained that while her parents had told her she was safe—and she trusted them—she felt alone and did not know what was happening (personal communication, December 31, 2015). Her lack of information made the situation fearful.

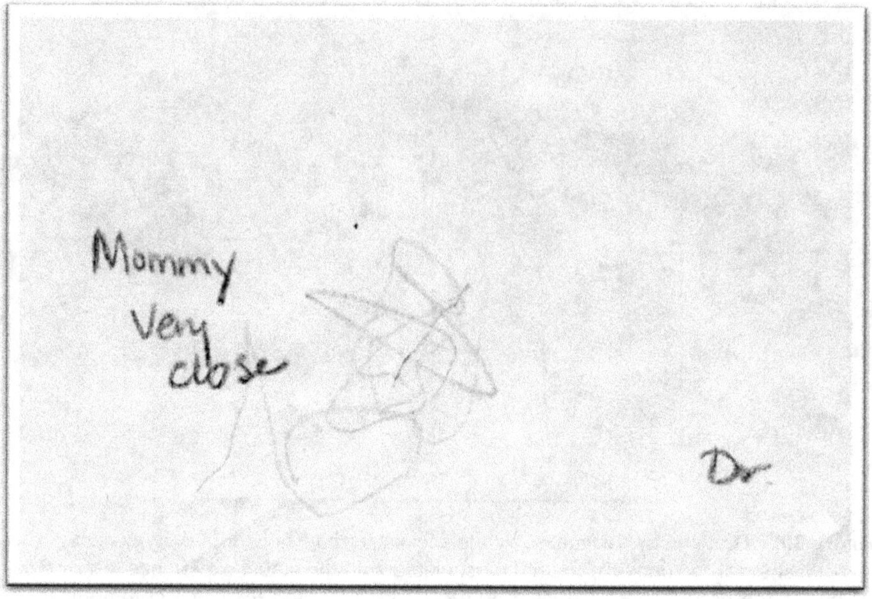

Figure B.10 Drawing by Victor, 3. While his fine motor skills have yet to develop, Victor attempted to draw himself in the hospital. As he drew, he described his picture and his comments were noted. Victor was very adamant about keeping his mother as close to him as possible while the doctor remained as far away as possible (personal communication, January 5, 2016). Not only is his effort to create consonance significant, his depiction of the affect his mother has is significant as well.

References

Adler, P. A. & Adler, P. (1997). Parent-as-researcher: The politics of researching in the personal life. In R. Hertz (Ed.), *Reflexivity and voice* (21–44). Thousand Oaks, CA: Sage Publications.

Agbenyega, J. S. (2014). Beyond alienation: Unpacking the methodological issues in visual research with children. In M. Fleer & A. Ridgway (Eds.). *Visual methodologies and digital tools for researching with young children* (153–168). Switzerland: Springer International Publishing.

Ahmad, R., Ferlie, E., & Atun, R. (2013). How trustworthiness is assessed in health-care: A sense-making perspective. *Journal of Change Management, 13* 13(2), 159–178.

Alderfer, M. A., Wiebe, D. J., & Hartmann, D. P. (2001). Social behaviour and illness information interact to influence the peer acceptance of children with chronic illness. *British Journal of Health Psychology, 6*, 243–255.

Alexander, A., Benjamin, L. M., Hoerrner, K., & Roe, D. (1998). "We'll be back in a moment": A content analysis of advertisements in children's television in the 1950s. *Journal of Advertising, 27*(3), 1–9.

Alfieri, L., Brooks, P. J., Aldrich, N. J., & Tenenbaum, H. R. (2011). Does discovery-based instruction enhance learning? *Journal of Educational Psychology*, 103, 1–18.

Anning, A. & Ring, K. (2004). *Making sense of children's drawings.* Maidenhead, UK: Open University Press.

Ashton-Shaeffer, C., Gibson, H. J., Autry, C. E., & Hanson, C. S. (2001). Meaning of sport to adults with physical disabilities: A disability sport camp experience. *Sociology of Sport Journal, 18*(1), 95–114.

Atkinson, R. (1998). *The life story interview.* Thousand Oaks, CA: Sage Publications, Inc.

Bandura, A. (1971). *Social learning theory.* New York: General Learning Press.

Bandura, A. (1982). Self-efficacy mechanism in human agency. *American Psychologist, 37*(2), 122–147.

Bandura, A. (2001). Social cognitive theory of mass communication. *Media Psychology, 3,* 265–299.

Beck, C. S. (2005). Becoming the story: Narratives as collaborative, social enactments of individual, relational, and public identities. In L. M. Harter, P. M. Japp, & C. S. Beck (Eds.), *Narratives, health, and healing: Communication theory, research, and practice* (61–82). Mahwah, NJ: Lawrence Erlbaum Associates, Publishers.

Bernard, H. R. (2006). *Research methods in anthropology: Qualitative and quantitative approaches* (4th ed.). Lanham, MD: AltaMira Press.

Bettelheim, B. (2010). *The uses of enchantment: The meaning and importance of fairy tales.* New York: Vintage Books. (Original work published 1975).

Beyer, J. M. (1992). Researchers are not cats: They can survive and succeed by being curious. In P. J. Frost & R. E. Stablein (Eds.). *Doing exemplary research* (65–72). Thousand Oaks, CA: Sage Publications.

Bickham, D. S., Vandewater, E. A., Huston, A. C., Lee, J. H., Caplovitz, A. G., Wright, J. C. (2009). Predictors of children's electronic media use: An examination of three ethnic groups. *Media Psychology, 5*(2), 107–137.

Bio. (2014). Fred Rogers biography. Retrieved from http://www.biography.com/people/fred-rogers-9462161#synopsis

Blount, R. L., Powers, S. W., Cotter, M. W., Swan, S., & Free, K. (1994). Making the system work: Training pediatric oncology patients to cope and their parents to coach them during BMAILP procedures. *Behavior Modification, 18*(1), 6–31.

Blum, N., Williams, G., Friman, P. C., & Christophersen, E. R. (1995). Disciplining young children: The role of reason. *Pediatrics,* 96, 336–341.

Bogden, R., Biklen, D., Shapiro, A., & Spelkoman, D. (1982). The disabled: Media's monster. *Social Policy, 13*(2), 32–35.

Bowlby, J. (1982). *Attachment and loss. Vol. 1: Attachment* (2nd ed.). New York: Basic Books (Original work published 1969).

Braithwaite, D. O. & Harter, L. M. (2000). Communication and the management of dialectical tensions in the personal relationships of people with disabilities. In D. O. Braithwaite and T. L. Thompson (Eds.). *Handbook of communication and people with disabilities: Research and application* (17–36). Mahway, NJ: Lawrence Erlbaum Associates.

Broome, M. E. (1986). The relationship between children's fears and behavior during a painful event. *Children's Health Care, 14*(3), 142–145.

Brown, A. D., Stacey, P., & Nandhakumar, J. (2008). Making sense of sense-making narratives. *Human Relations, 61*(8), 1035–1062.

Brown, P. (2006). Children of the revolution: The making of young citizens. *Modern & Contemporary France,* 14(2), 205–220.

Brown, W. J. & Singhal, A. (1999). Entertainment-education strategies for social change. In D. P. Demers & K. Viswanath (Eds.). *Mass media, social control and social change: A macrosocial perspective* (263–280). Ames, IA: Iowa State University Press.

Bruner, J. (1986). *Actual minds, possible worlds.* Cambridge, MA: Harvard University Press.

Bruner, J. & Haste, H. (2011). *Making sense: The child's construction of the world.* New York: Routledge.

Buckingham, D. (1993). *Reading audiences: Young people and the media.* Manchester, NY: Manchester University Press.

Buckingham, D. (2000). *After the death of childhood: Growing up in the age of electronic media.* Cambridge, UK: Polity Press

Buckingham, D. (2003). *Media education: Literacy, learning, and contemporary culture.* Cambridge, UK: Polity Press.

Buckingham, D. (2007). Childhood in the age of global media. *Children's Geographies, 5(1/2)*, 43–54.

Buckingham, D. & Sefton-Green, J. (2004). Gotta catch 'em all: Structure, agency, and pedagogy in children's media culture. In J. Tobin (Ed.). *Pikachu's global adventure: The rise and fall of Pokemon* (12–33). Durham, NC: Duke University Press.

Burke, K. (1973). *The philosophy of literary form: Studies in symbolic action.* Berkeley, CA: University of California Press.

Carabas, T. & Harter, L. M. (2005). State-induced illness and forbidden stories: The role of storytelling in healing individual and social traumas in Romania. In L. M. Harter, P. M. Japp, & C. S. Beck (Eds.). *Narratives, health, and healing: Communication theory, research, and practice* (149–168). Mahwah, NJ: Lawrence Erlbaum Associates, Publishers.

Champion, M., Noettes, A. D., Taboulet, P., & Lemerle, S. (1999). Secrecy in children with HIV infection. *Archives de Pediatrie, 6*(10), 1101–1108.

Charon, R. (2006). *Narrative medicine: Honoring the stories of illness.* New York: Oxford University Press.

Chew, K. (2008). Disabilities and the media. In R. Andersen & J. Gray (Eds.), *Battleground: The media* (Vol. 2, 123–129). Westport, CT: Greenwood Press.

Cohen, L. L., Bernard, R. S., Greco, L. A., & McClellan, C. B. (2002). A child-focused intervention for coping with procedural pain: Are parent and nurse coaches necessary? *Journal of Pediatric Psychology, 27*(8), 749–757.

Cohen, M. (2012). The role of research and evaluation in educational media. In D. G. Singer & J. L. Singer (Eds.). *Handbook of children and the media* (2nd ed., 527–551). Thousand Oaks, CA: Sage Publications.

Coles, R. (1990). *The spiritual life of children.* Boston, MA: Houghton Mifflin Company.

Collins, D. (2004, January 23). 'Captain Kangaroo' dead at 76. *CBSNews.* Retrieved from http://www.cbsnews.com/news/captain-kangaroo-dead-at-76/

Comber, B. (2013). Schools as meeting places: Critical and inclusive literacies in changing local environments. *Language Arts, 90*(5), 361–371.

Comstock, G. & Sharrer, E. (2012). Use of television and other media. In D. G. Singer & J. L. Singer (Eds.), *Handbook of children and media* (2nd ed., 13–44). Thousand Oaks, CA: Sage Publications.

Corsaro, W. A. (2005). *The sociology of childhood* (2nd ed.). London, UK: Sage Publications.

Coulehan, J. (1991). The word as an instrument of healing. *Literature and Medicine, 18*, 111–129.

Covey, H. C. (1998). *Social perceptions of people with disabilities in history.* Springfield, IL: Charles C. Thomas.

Craddock, F. B. (2002). *Overhearing the gospel.* St. Louis, MO: Chalice Press.

Davidson, J. E. (2010). Facilitated sense-making: A strategy and new middle-range theory to support families of intensive care unit patients. *Critical Care Nurse, 30*(6), 28–39.

Denzin, N. K., & Lincoln, Y. S. (2003). Introduction: The discipline and practice of qualitative research. In N. K. Denzin & Y. S. Lincoln (Eds.), *The landscape of qualitative research: Theories and issues* (2nd ed., 1–46). Thousand Oaks, Sage Publications, Inc.

Dervin, B. (1983, May). *An Overview of Sense-Making Research: Concepts, Methods and Results.* Paper presented at the annual meeting of the International Communication Association, Dallas, TX. Available: http://communication.sbs.ohio-state.edu/sense-making/art/artdervin83.html

Dervin, B. (1992). From the mind's eye of the user: The Sense-Making qualitative-quantitative methodology. In J. D. Glazier & R. R. Powell (Eds.). *Qualitative research in information management* (61–84). Englewood, CO: Libraries Unlimited.

Dervin, B. (2003a). Audience as listener and learner, teacher and confidante: The Sense-Making approach. In B. Dervin, L. Foreman-Wernet, & E. Lauterbach (Eds.). *Sense-Making methodology reader: Selected writings of Brenda Dervin* (215–232). Cresskill, NJ: Hampton Press, Inc.

Dervin, B. (2003b). A theoretic perspective and research approach for generating research helpful to communication practice. In B. Dervin, L. Foreman-Wernet, & E. Lauterbach (Eds.). *Sense-Making methodology reader: Selected writings of Brenda Dervin* (251–268). Cresskill, NJ: Hampton Press, Inc.

Dervin, B. (2003c). Verbing communication: Mandate for disciplinary invention. In B. Dervin, L. Foreman-Wernet, & E. Lauterbach (Eds.). *Sense-Making methodology reader: Selected writings of Brenda Dervin* (101–109). Cresskill, NJ: Hampton Press, Inc.

Dervin, B. (2008). *Interviewing as dialectical practice: Sense-Making Methodology as exemplar.* Paper presented to the annual meeting of International Association for Media and Communication Research. Stockholm, Sweden. July 2008.

Dervin, B., Foreman-Wernet, L., & Lauterbach, E. (Eds.). (2003). *Sense-making methodology reader: Selected writings of Brenda Dervin.* Cresskill, NJ: Hampton Press, Inc.

Diem-Wille, G. (2001). A therapeutic perspective: The use of drawings in child psychoanalysis and social science. In T. V. Leeuwen & C. Jewitt (Eds.). *Handbook of visual analysis* (119–133). Thousand Oaks, CA: Sage Publications.

Du, S., Jaaniste, T., Champion, G. D., & Yap, C. S. L. (2008). Theories of fear acquisition: The development of needle phobia in children. *Pediatric Pain Letter: Commentaries on Pain in Infants, Children, and Adolescents, 10*(2), 13–17.

Duggan, A., Bradshaw, Y. S., & Altman, W. (2010). How do I ask about your disability? An examination of interpersonal communication processes between medical students and patients with disabilities. *Journal of Health Communication*, 15(3), 334–350.

Eilertsen, M. B., Kristiansen, K., Reinfjell, T., Rannestad, T., Indredavik, M. S., & Vik, T. (2009). Professional collaboration—support for children with cancer and their families—focus group interview—a source of information and knowledge—professionals' perspectives. *Journal of Interprofessional Care, 23*(4), 355–368.

Ellis, R. & Leventhal, B. (1993). Information needs and decision-making preferences of children with cancer. *Psycho-Oncology, 2,* 277–284.

Endacott, J.L. & Bowles, F.A. (2013). Avoiding the 'It's a Small World' effect: A lesson plan to explore diversity. *Multicultural Education 20*(2), 43–48.

Erickson, M. F., Sroufe, L. A., & Egeland, B. (1985). The relationship between quality of attachment and behavior problems in preschool in a high-risk sample. *Monographs of the Society for Research in Child Development, 50*(1), 147–166.

Evans, C.S. (1982). *Subjectivity and religious belief.* Washington, DC: University Press of America.

Fernandes, S. C., Arriaga, P., & Esteves, F. (2014). Providing preoperative information for children undergoing surgery: a randomized study testing different types of education material to reduce children's preoperative worries. *Health Education Research, 29*(6), 1058–1076.

Festinger, L. (1957). *A theory of cognitive dissonance.* Stanford, CA: Stanford University Press.

Fiedler, L. (1978). *Freaks: Myths and images of the secret self.* New York: Simon and Schuster.

Field, A. P. (2006). The behavioral inhibition system and the verbal information pathway to children's fears. *Journal of Abnormal Psychology, 115*(4), 742–752

Fine, M., & Asch, A. (1988). Disability beyond stigma: Social interaction, discrimination, and activism. *Journal of Social Issues, 44,* 3–21.

Fink, A. (2003). *The survey handbook.* Thousand Oaks, CA: Sage Publications.

Fisher, K. R., Hirsh-Pasek, K., Newcombe, N., & Golinkoff, R. M. (2013). Taking shape: Supporting preschoolers' acquisition of geometric knowledge through guided play. *Child Development, 84*(6), 1872–1878.

Folkman, S. (2008). The case for positive emotions in the stress process. *Anxiety, Stress, and Coping, 21*(1), 3–14.

Frank, A. W. (1995). *The wounded storyteller: Body, illness, and ethics.* Chicago, IL: University of Chicago Press.

Frank, A. W. (2001). *Acts of witness: Forms of engagement in illness.* Presentation at narrative based medicine conference, 3 September, Cambridge, UK.

Fraser, B. P. & Brown, W. J. (2002). Media, celebrities, and social influence: Identification with Elvis Presley. *Mass Communication and Society, 5*(2), 183–206.

Freud, S. (1920). *A general introduction to psychoanalysis* (G. S. Hall, Trans.). New York: Boni and Liveright. Retrieved from http://www.bartleby.com/283/

Fury, G., Carlson, E., & Sroufe, A. (1997). Children's representations of attachment relationships in family drawings. *Child Development, 68*(6), 1154–1164.

Gardner, H. (1980). *Artful scribbles: The significance of children's drawings.* New York: Basic Books.

Giddens, A. (1991). *Modernity and self identity.* Stanford, CA: Stanford University Press.

Gillis, A. J. (1990). Hospital preparation: The children's story. *Children's Health Care, 19*(1), 19–27.

Goetze, G. & Myers-Walls, J. (2013). Ways to help children cope with their fears. *Provider-Parent Partnerships.* Retrieved from https://www.extension.purdue.edu/providerparent/child%20growth-development/Ways_Help_Cope_Fears.htm

Goffman, E. (1967). *Interaction ritual: Essays on face-to-face behavior.* Garden City, NY: Anchor Books.

Goodall, H. L., Jr. (2000). *Writing the new ethnography.* New York: Altmira Press.

Griswold, W. (1994). *Cultures and societies in a changing world.* Thousand Oaks, CA: Sage Publications.

Grose, M. (2013). Helping kids be brave. Retrieved from http://www.parentingideas.com.au/Blog/April-2013-(1)/Raising-kids-to-be-brave-(and-not-anxious)

Guillemin, M. (2004). Heart disease and mid-age women: Focusing on gender and age. *Health Sociology Review, 13*(1), 7–14.

Gurian, M. & Ballew, A. C. (2003). *The boys and girls learn differently: Action guide for teachers.* San Francisco, CA: Jossey-Bass.

Hampel, P., Rudolph, H., Rainer, S., Lab-Lentzsch, A., & Petermann, F. (2005). Coping among children and adolescents with chronic illness. *Anxiety, Stress, and Coping, 18*(2), 145–155.Harter, L. (2013). *Imagining new normals: A narrative framework for health communication.* Dubuque, IA: Kendall Hunt Publishing Company.

Hayden, S. (1993). Chronically ill and 'feeling fine': A study of communication and chronic illness. *Journal of Applied Communication Research, 21*(3), 263–278.

Hodkinson, P. (2002). *Goth: Identity, style and subculture.* Oxford, UK: Berg.

Hogan, M. J. (2012). Parents and other adults: Models and monitors of healthy media habits. In D. G. Singer & J. L. Singer (Eds.). *Handbook of children and the media* (2nd ed., 661–680). Thousand Oaks, CA: Sage Publications.

Hollenbeck, A. R. & Slaby, R. G. (1979). Infant visual and vocal responses to television. *Child Development, 50,* 41–45.

Honomichl, R. D., & Chen, Z. (2012). The role of guidance in children's discovery learning. *WIREs Cognitive Science*, 3, 615–622.

Hooker, L. (1997). Information needs of teenagers with cancer: Developing a tool to explore the perceptions of patients and professionals. *Journal of Cancer Nursing, 1*(4), 160–168.

Hudson, J. L. & Rapee, R. M. (2001). Parent-child interactions and anxiety disorders: An observational study. *Behaviour Research and Therapy, 39*, 1411–1427.

Hunt, S. B. (2003). An essay on publishing standards for rhetorical criticism. *Communication Studies, 53*(3), 378–384.

Huntemann, N. & Morgan, M. (2012). Media and identity development. In D. G. Singer & J. L. Singer (Eds.). *Handbook of children and the media* (2nd ed., 303–319). Thousand Oaks, CA: Sage Publications.

Hurst, C., Corning, K., & Ferrante, R. (2012). Children's acceptance of others with disability: The influence of a disability-simulation program. *Journal of Genetic Counseling*, *21*(6), 873–883.

Jaaniste, T., Hayes, B. K., & von Baeyer, C. L. (2007). Providing children with information about forthcoming medical procedures: A review and synthesis. *Clinical Psychology Science and Practice, 14*(2), 124–143.

Janks, H. (2010). *Literacy and power*. London, UK: Routledge.

Jansen, H. (2010). The logic of qualitative survey research and its position in the field of social research methods. *Forum Qualitative Sozialforschung, 11*(2), 11.

Japp, P. M., Harter, L. M., & Beck, C. S. (2005). Overview of narrative and health communication theorizing. In L. M. Harter, P. M. Japp, & C. S. Beck (Eds.), *Narratives, health, and healing: Communication theory, research, and practice* (1–6). Mahwah, NJ: Lawrence Erlbaum Associates, Publishers.

Jones, T. W., Sowell, V. M., Jones, J. K., & Butler, L. G. (1981). Changing children's perceptions of handicapped people. *Exceptional Children, 47*(5), 365–368.

Kaiser Family Foundation. (2010). *Daily media use among children and teens up dramatically from five years ago.* Retrieved from http://kff.org/disparities-policy/press-release/daily-media-use-among-children-and-teens-up-dramatically-from-five-years-ago/

Kalitzkus, V. & Matthiessen, P. F. (2009). Narrative-based medicine: Potential, pitfalls, and practice. *The Permanente Journal, 13*(1), 80–86.

Kean, S. (2009). Children and young people's strategies to access information during a family member's critical illness. *Journal of Clinical Nursing, 19,* 266–274.

Kendrick, M. & McKay, R. (2004). Drawings as an alternative way of understanding young children's construction of literacy. *Journal of Early Childhood Literacy, 4*(1), 109–128.

Kennedy, C. E., Moore, P. J., Peterson, R. A., Katzman, M. A., Vermani, M., &Charmak, W. D. (2011). What makes people anxious about pain? How personality and perception combine to determine pain anxiety responses in clinical and non-clinical populations. *Anxiety, Stress, and Coping, 24*(2), 179–200.

Kierkegaard, S. (1992). *Concluding unscientific postscript to philosophical fragments* (Vol. 1) (Hong, H., & Hong, E., Trans.). Princeton, NJ: Princeton University Press. (Original work published 1846).

Kierkegaard, S. (2003). *Fear and trembling* (A. Hannay, Trans.). New York: Penguin Group. (Original work published 1843).

King, N. J., Heyne, D., Gullone, E., & Molloy, G. N. (2001). Usefulness of emotive imagery in the treatment of childhood phobias: Clinical guidelines, case examples and issues. *Counseling Psychology Quarterly, 14*(2), 95–101.

Kinnunen, S. & Einarsdottir, J. (2013). Feeling, wondering, sharing and constructing life: Aesthetic experience and life changes in young children's drawing stories. *International Journal of Early Childhood, 45,* 359–385.

Klefstad, J. & Martinez, K. (2013). Using multicultural children's literature to promote cultural awareness and appreciation. *Young Children, 68*(5), 74–81.

Klingman, A., Melamed, B. G., Cuthbert, M. I., & Hermecz, D. A. (1984). Effects of participant modeling on information acquisition and skill utilization. *Journal of Consulting and Clinical Psychology, 52*(3), 414–422.

Koppers, S., & Cato, B. A. (2008). Trivialization is not a trivial means of dissonance reduction. Paper presented at the Psi Chi Regional Undergraduate Research Competition, Kansas City, MO.

Kress, G., & Jewitt, C. (2003). Introduction. In C. Jewitt & G. Kress (Eds.), *Multimodal literacy* (1–18). New York: Peter Lang.

Kuhn, A. (1985). *The power of the image.* London, UK: Routledge.

La Greca, A. M. & Bearman, K. J. (2000). Commentary: Children with pediatric conditions: Can peers' impressions be managed? And what about their friends? *Journal of Pediatric Psychology, 25*(3), 147–149.

Ladd, G. (1992). Themes and theories: Perspectives on processes in family-peer relationships. In R. Parke & D. Ladd (Eds.), *Family-peer relationships: Modes of linkage* (1–34). Hillsdale, NJ: Lawrence Erlbaum.

Lane, H. (1992). *The mask of benevolence: Disabling the deaf community.* New York: Alfred A. Knopf.

Langer, D. A., Chen, E., Luhmann, J. D. (2005). Attributions and coping in children's pain experiences. *Journal of Pediatric Psychology, 30(7), 615–622.*

Lauricella, A. R., Gola, A. A. H., & Calvert, S. L. (2011). Toddlers' learning from socially meaningful video characters. *Media Psychology, 14*, 216–232.

Le Goff, J. (1990). *Medieval history: 400–1500.* New York: Basil Blackwell.

Leitch, R. (2008). Creatively researching children's narratives through images and drawings. In P. Thomson (Ed.), *Doing visual research with children and young people* (37–58). London, UK: Routledge.

Leroy, S., Elixson, M., O'Brien, P., Tong, E., Turpin, S., & Usark, K. (2003). Recommendations for preparing children and adolescents for invasive cardiac procedures: A statement from the American Heart Association Pediatric Nursing Subcommittee of the Council on Cardiovascular Nursing in collaboration with the Council on Cardiovascular Diseases of the Young. *American Heart Association.* Retrieved from http://circ.ahajournals.org/content/108/20/2550

Levin, D. (2010). Remote control childhood: Combating the hazards of media culture in schools. *New Horizons in Education, 58*(3), 14–25.

Liamputtong, P. & Fernandes, S. (2015). What makes people sick? The drawing method and children's conceptualization of health and illness. *Australasian Journal of Early Childhood, 40*(1), 23–31.

Libresco, A. S., Balantic, J., & Kipling, J.C. (2011). *Every book is a social studies book: How to meet standards with picture books, K–6.* Santa Barbara, CA: ABC-CLIO.

Lichty, L. & Topping, M. (1975). *American broadcasting.* New York: Hastings House.

Lincoln, Y.S. & Guba, E. G. (1985). *Naturalistic Inquiry.* Thousand Oaks, CA: Sage Publications.

Lohause, A., Ball, J., Klein-Hessling, J., & Wild, M. (2005). Relations between media use and self-reported symptomatology in young adolescents. *Anxiety, Stress, and Coping, 18*(4), 333–341.

Longhin, L. (2011). Psychic-mental suffering. *Contemporary Psychoanalytic Studies, 13*, 91–117.

Lovelace, V. & Huston, H. C. (1983). Can television teach prosocial behavior? *Prevention in Human Services, 2*, 93–106.

Luke, A. (2012). Critical literacy: Foundational notes. *Theory into Practice, 51*(1), 4–11.

MacIntyre, A. (1981). *After virtue: A study in moral theory.* Notre Dame, IN: University of Notre Dame Press.

MacQuarrie, J. (2012, April 12). Doc McStuffins and writer-producer Chris Nee. *Wired.* Retrieved from http://www.wired.com/geekdad/2012/05/doc-mcstuffins-and-writer-producer-chris-nee/

Mahajan, L., Wyllie, R., Steffen, R., Kay, M., Kitaoka, G., Dettorre, J., et al. (1998). The effects of a psychological preparation program on anxiety in children and adolescents undergoing gastrointestinal endoscopy. *Journal of Pediatric Gastroenterology & Nutrition*, 27(2), 161–165.

Mantei, J. & Kervin, L. (2015). Examining the interpretations children share from their reading of an almost wordless picture book during independent reading time. *Australian Journal of Language & Literacy*, 38(3), 183–192.

Mares, M. & Woodard, E. H. (2012). Effects of prosocial media content on children's social interactions. In D. G. Singer & J. L. Singer (Eds.). *Handbook of children and the media* (2nd ed., 197–214). Thousand Oaks, CA: Sage Publications.

Matthews, C. K. & Harrington, N. G. (2000). Invisible disability. In D. O. Braithwaite and T. L. Thompson (Eds.). *Handbook of communication and people with disabilities: Research and application* (405–423). Mahway, NJ: Lawrence Erlbaum Associates.

McGee, M. C. (1980). The "ideograph": A link between rhetoric and ideology. *The Quarterly Journal of Speech, 66*(1), 1–16.

McKay, R. A. & Kendrick, M. E. (2001). Children draw their images of reading and writing. *Language Arts, 78*(6), 529–533.

McLuhan, M. (1964). *Understanding media: The extension of man.* London, UK: Routledge.

Melamed, B. G., Dearborn, M., & Hermecz, D. A. (1983). Necessary considerations for surgery preparation: Age and previous experience. *Psychosomatic Medicine, 45*(6), 517–525.

Melamed, B. G., Meyer, R., Gee, C., & Soule, L. (1976). The influence of time and type of preparation on children's adjustment to hospitalization. *Journal of Pediatric Psychology, 1,* 31–37.

Melendez, L. (2015). Using children's books as a social studies curriculum strategy. *Young Children,* 48–53.

Meltzoff, A. N. (1988). Imitation of televised models by infants. *Child Development, 59,* 1221–1229.

Merleau-Ponty, M. (2010). *Child psychology and pedagogy the Sorbonne lectures 1949–1952.* Translated from the French by Talia Welsh. Evanston, IL: Northwestern University Press. [Original book: *Psychologie et pedagogie de l'enfant: Cours de Sorbonne 1949–1952*, Editions Verdier, 2001].

Merriam, S. B. (2002). Basic interpretive qualitative research. In S. B. Merriam (Ed.),*Qualitative research in practice: Examples for discussion and analysis* (37–39). San Francisco, CA: Jossey-Bass.

Meyerson, L. (1948). Physical disability as a social psychological problem. *Journal of Social Issues*, 4(4), 2–10.

Mishler, E. G. (1986). *Research interviewing: Context and narrative.* Cambridge, MA: Harvard University Press.

Mitchell, W. (2012). Making choices about medical interventions: The experience of disabled young people with degenerative conditions. *Health Expectations, 17,* 254–266.

Mitchell W, Clarke S, Sloper P. (2006). Care and support needs of children and young people with cancer and their parents. *Psycho-Oncology*, *15*, 805–816.

Monbeck, M. E. (1973). *The meaning of blindness: Attitudes toward blindness and blind people.* Bloomington, IN: Indiana University Press.

Montgomery, K. (2013). *How doctors think: Clinical judgment and the practice of medicine.* Oxford, UK: Oxford University Press.

Muris, P., Merckelbach, H., Ollendick, T. H., King, N. J., & Bogie, N. (2001). Children's nighttime fears: parent-child ratings of frequency, content, origins, coping behaviors and severity. *Behavior Research and Therapy, 39*, 13–28.

Nielsen, K. E. (2012). *A disability history of the United States.* Boston, MA: Beacon Press.

Oakley, A., Bendelow, G., Barnes, J., Buchanan, M., & Husain, O. (1995). Health and cancer prevention: Knowledge and beliefs of children and young people. *British Medical Journal, 310*(6986), 1029–1033.

O'Connor, F. (1979). *Letters of Flannery O'Connor: The habit of being.* S. Fitzgerald (Ed.). New York: The Noonday Press.

Ollendick, T. H., & King, N. J. (1991). Origins of childhood fears: an evaluation of Rachman's theory of fear acquisition. *Behaviour Research and Therapy*, 29, 117–123.

Ong, W. J. (2002). *Orality and literacy.* New York: Routledge.

Osborn, M. (1967). Archetypal metaphor in rhetoric: The light-dark family. *Quarterly Journal of Speech, 53*(2), 115–126.

Parsloe, S. M. (2015). Discourses of disability, narratives of community: Reclaiming an autistic identity online. *Journal of Applied Communication Research,* 43(3), 336–356.

Patton, M. Q. (2002). *Qualitative research and evaluation methods* (3rd ed.). Thousand Oaks, CA: Sage Publications.

Pinto, R. P. & Hollandsworth, Jr., J. G. (1989). Using videotape modeling to prepare children psychologically for surgery: Influence of parents and costs versus benefits of providing preparation services. *Health Psychology, 8*(1), 79–95.

Pouchelle, M. C. (1990). *The body and surgery in the Middle Ages,* trans. Rosemary Morris. Cambridge, UK: Polity Press.

Potter, J. (2005). Making psychology relevant. *Discourse & Society, 16*(5), 739–747.

Pouchelle, M. C. (1990). *The body and surgery in the Middle Ages.* New Brunswick, NJ: Rutgers University Press.

Prosser, J. (1998). The status of image-based research. In J. Prosser (Ed.), *Image-based research: A sourcebook for qualitative researchers* (97–112). London, UK: Falmer.

Randles, D., Inzlicht, M., Proulx, T., Tullet, A. M., & Heine, S. J. (2015). Is dissonance reduction a special case of fluid compensation? Evidence that dissonant cognitions cause compensatory affirmation and abstraction. *Journal of Personality and Social Psychology, 108*(5), 697–710.

Ricoeur, P. (1998). Philosophy after Kierkegaard. In J. Ree & J. Chamberlain (Eds.), *Kierkegaard: A critical reader* (9–25). Malden, MA: Blackwell Publishing.

Rideout, V. J. & Hamel, E. (2006). *The media family: Electronic media in the lives of infants, toddlers, preschoolers, and their parents.* Menlo Park, CA: Kaiser

Family Foundation. Retrieved from https://kaiserfamilyfoundation.files.wordpress.com/2013/01/7500.pdf

Rideout, V. J., Vandewater, E. A., & Wartella, E.A. (2003). *Zero to Six: Electronic Media in the Lives of Infants, Toddlers, and Preschoolers.* Menlo Park, CA: Kaiser Family Foundation. Retrieved from http://files.eric.ed.gov/fulltext/ED482302.pdf

Riessman, C. K. (2008). *Narrative methods for the human sciences.* Thousand Oaks, CA: Sage Publications.

Rubin, A. M. (2009). Uses-and-gratifications perspective on media effects. In B. Jennings & M. B. Oliver (Eds.), *Media effects: Advances in theory and research* (3rd ed., 165–178). New York: Routledge.

Saint-Loup, A. (1993). Images of the deaf in medieval western Europe. In Fisher, R. & Lane, H. (Eds.). *Looking back: A reader on the history of the deaf communities and their sign languages* (379–402). Hamburg, Germany: Signum.

Salmela, M., Salantera, S., Ruotsalainen, T., & Aronen, E. T. (2010). Coping strategies for hospital-related fears in pre-school-aged children. *Journal of Paediatrics and Child Health,* 46, 108–114.

Sambuchino, C. (2010, March 3). Writing tips from Max Lucado, best-selling author. Retrieved from http://www.writersdigest.com/editor-blogs/guide-to-literary-agents/writing-tips-from-max-lucado-best-selling-author

Scheer, J. & Groce, N. (1988). Impairment as a human constant: Cross-cultural and historical perspectives on variation. *Journal of Social Issues,* 44(1), 23–37.

Schmitt, K. L., Anderson, D. R., & Collins, P. A. (1999). Form and content: Looking at visual features of television. *Developmental Psychology,* 35, 1156–1167.

Scott, B. G. & Weems, C. F. (2010). Patterns of actual and perceived control: Are control profiles differentially related to internalizing and externalizing problems in youth? *Anxiety, Stress, and Coping,* 23(5), 515–528.

Seidman, I. (2006). *Interviewing as qualitative research: A guide for researchers in education and the social sciences* (3rd ed.). New York: Teachers College Press.

Sesame Workshop Family. (n.d.). *FAQs.* Retrieved from http://www.sesameworkshop.org/faqs/

Sheppard, P. (2012, October 3). Mickey Mouse Club: Reaching new generations 57 years later. *Disney Post: The Official Blog of The Walt Disney Company.* Retrieved from https://thewaltdisneycompany.com/blog/mickey-mouse-club-reaching-new-generations-57-years-later

Silverman, D. (2011). *Interpreting qualitative data* (4th ed.). London, UK: Sage Publications.

Simcock, G., Garrity, K., & Barr, R. (2011). The Effect of Narrative Cues on Infants' Imitation From Television and Picture Books. *Child Development, 82*(5), 1607–1619.

Soule, K. P. & Roloff, M. E. (2000). Help between persons with and without disabilities from a resource theory perspective. In D. O. Braithwaite and T. L. Thompson (Eds.). *Handbook of communication and people with disabilities: Research and application* (67–83). Mahway, NJ: Lawrence Erlbaum Associates.

Sposito, A. M. P., Silva-Rodrigues, F. M., Sparapani, V. D. C., Pfeifer, L. L., de Lima, R. A. G., Nascimento, L. C. (2015). Coping strategies used by hospitalized children with cancer undergoing chemotherapy. *Journal of Nursing Scholarship,* 47(2), 143–151.

Sterling, C. & Kittross, J. (1990). *Stay tuned: A concise history of American broadcasting.* Belmont, CA: Wadsworth.

Stets, J. E. & Burke, P. J. (2000). Identity theory and social identity theory. *Social Psychology Quarterly,* 63(3), 224–237.

Stilwell, H. (2015). *Helping children cope: Embracing the role and effectiveness of medically themed media.* Paper presented to the annual conference of the National Communication Association. Las Vegas, Nevada. November 2015.

Strong, D. A. & Brown, W. J. (2011). Promoting prosocial beliefs and behavior towards people with disabilities in Nepal through a children's entertainment-education program. *Disability, CBR & Inclusive Development, 22*(2), 22–37.

Strouse, G. A. & Troseth, G. L. (2008). "Don't try this at home": Toddler's imitation of new skills from people on video. *Journal of Experimental Child Psychology,* 101, 262–280.

Tajfel, H. (1978). The achievement of group differentiation. In H. Tajfel (Ed.), *Differentiation between social groups: Studies in the social psychology of intergroup relations* (77–98). London, UK: Academic Press.

Tajfel, H., & Turner, J. C. (1985). The social identity theory of intergroup behavior. In S. Worchel, & W. G. Austin (Ed.), *Psychology of intergroup relations* (2nd ed., 7–24). Chicago, IL: Nelson-Hall.

Taub, D. E., & Greer, K. R. (2000). Physical activity as a normalizing experience for school-age children with physical disabilities: Implications for legitimation of social identity and enhancement of social ties. *Journal of Sport & Social Issues,* 24(4), 395–414.

Taylor, C. C. W. (1976). *Plato, Protagoras.* Oxford, UK: Oxford University Press.

Taylor, S. J. & Bogdan, R. (1984). *Introduction to qualitative research methods: The search for meaning.* New York: John Wiley.

Tracy, S. J. (2013). *Qualitative research methods: Collecting evidence, crafting analysis, communicating impact.* Malden, MA: Wiley-Blackwell.

Valenti, K. (2013). The single most effective way to help children overcome fear. Retrieved from http://www.totthoughts.com/pebbles-of-bravery/

Van Gorp, B. (2007). The constructionist approach to framing: Bringing culture back in. *Journal of Communication,* 57, 60–78.

Vierhaus, M., Lohaus, A., & Ball, J. (2007). Developmental changes in coping: Situational and methodological influences. *Anxiety, Stress, and Coping*, 20(3), 267–282.

Vygotsky, L. (1997). Interaction between learning and development. In M. Gauvain & M. Cole (Eds.). *Readings on the development of children* (2nd ed., 29–36). New York: W. H. Freeman and Company.

Wakefield, J. C. (1992). Freud and the intentionality of affect. *Psychoanalytic Psychology, 9*(1), 1–23.

Warren, M. (1997). *Seeing through the media: A religious view of communications and cultural analysis.* Harrisburg, PA: Trinity Press International.

Waska, R. (2012). Entitled and demanding. *Contemporary Psychoanalytic Studies,* 17, 13–29.

Watson, D. L. & Emery C. (2010). From rhetoric to reality: The problematic nature and assessment of children and young people's social and emotional learning. *British Educational Research Journal,* 36(5), 767–786.

Weber, H. (2003). Breaking the rules: Personal and social responses to coping norm-violations. *Anxiety, Stress, and Coping,* 16(2), 133–153.

Westphal, M. (1996). *Becoming a self: A reading of Kierkegaard's concluding unscientific postscript.* West Lafayette, IN: Purdue University Press.

Whiting, M. (2009). *"Is this my life?": Meaning and sense-making as key determinants of parents' experience when caring for children with disabilities, life-threatening/life-limiting illness or technology dependence* (Doctoral dissertation). Retrieved from British Library EThOs, EBSCOhost (306.874).

Wilson, B. (2008). Media and children's aggression, fear, and altruism. *Children and Electronic Media, 18*(1), 87–118.

Zangori, L. & Forbes, C. T. (2013). Preservice elementary teachers and explanation construction: Knowledge-for-practice and knowledge-in-practice. *Science Education, 97*(2), 310–330.

Zola, I. K. (1993). Self, identity, and the naming question: Reflections of the language of disability. *Society, Science, & Medicine, 36,* 167–173.

Index

About the Author

Heather A. Stilwell was born and raised in Southern California learning to love listening to and telling other people's stories. She began a broadcast journalism career that took her to the East Coast and the Midwest before returning home to be closer to her family while expecting her first child. She has a PhD in communication from Regent University. Heather and her husband, Steve, are currently living in Southern California with their three children. Their family medical experiences are the inspiration behind her research. When not writing and researching, Heather enjoys spending time at the ice rink, exploring nature with her children, and creating art.

About the Author

www.ingramcontent.com/pod-product-compliance
Lightning Source LLC
LaVergne TN
LVHW011519200926
848484LV00001B/70
* 9 7 8 1 4 9 8 5 5 1 9 8 4 *